A Very
Strange Man

OTHER BOOKS BY ALANNAH HOPKIN

Fiction and Short Stories
A Joke Goes a Long Way in the Country (1982)
The Out-haul (1985)
The Dogs of Inishere (2017)

Non-fiction
The Living Legend of St Patrick (1989)
Inside Cork: An Independent Guide (1992)
Eating Scenery: West Cork, the People and the Place (2008)
The Ship of Seven Murders: A True Story of Madness and Murder (2010; with Kathy Bunney)
On the Banks: Cork City in Poems and Songs (2016; editor)

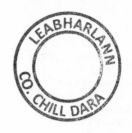

ALANNAH HOPKIN

A Very Strange Man

A Memoir of Aidan Higgins

NEW ISLAND

A VERY STRANGE MAN
First published in 2021 by
New Island Books
Glenshesk House
10 Richview Office Park
Clonskeagh
Dublin D14 V8C4
Republic of Ireland

www.newisland.ie

Print ISBN: 978-1-84840-793-0
eBook ISBN: 978-1-84840-794-7

Typeset by JVR Creative India
Cover design by New Island Books
Edited by Bill Swainson
Printed by ScandBook, scandbook.com

New Island received financial assistance from The Arts Council (An Chomhairle Ealaíon), Dublin, Ireland.

New Island Books is a member of Publishing Ireland.

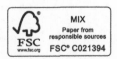

MIX
Paper from
responsible sources
FSC® C021394
www.fsc.org

For Carl, Julien and Elwin

In memory of Aidan Higgins
3 March 1927–27 December 2015

Aidan Higgins is a very strange man.
JOHN CALDER

I am consumed by memories and they form the life of me; stories that make up my life and lend it whatever veracity and purpose it may have.
AIDAN HIGGINS, *Donkey's Years*

Long ago I was this, was that, twisting and turning, incredulous, baffled, believing nothing, believing all. Now I am, what? I feel frightened, sometimes, but may be just tired. I feel depressed quite often, but may be just hungry.
All but blind
In his chambered hole
Gropes for worms...
AIDAN HIGGINS, *Scenes from a Receding Past*

CONTENTS

PREFACE

This is a memoir of the years that I spent living with the writer Aidan Higgins. I did not want to write a biography, nor a work of literary criticism. I wanted to write the book that only I could write, an account of his life from the age of fifty-nine, when we first met, to his death twenty-nine years later.

Aidan was one of the great stylists of the late twentieth century, generally acknowledged as the true heir of James Joyce, Samuel Beckett and Flann O'Brien – a risk-taker, learned, jocular, bawdy, ironic, disdainful, unpredictable. He made up his own rules as a writer as he went along, abandoning the conventions of fiction for a multi-stranded form that combined autobiography, anecdote, letters, diaries, lists, quotations and essays in a whirlwind of words, the whole presided over by his authorial alter ego, Rory of the Hills. All his life he was obsessed by memory: 'Is the memory of things better than the things themselves?'

My aim was to shed what light I could on the books and other pieces that he wrote while we were together, and to describe his working methods. I also wanted to record watching someone you love develop and live with dementia, in the hope that what I learnt from that experience might be useful to others.

I soon realised that I would need to read Aidan's diaries and consult other papers of his that were now in the Harry

Ransom Center at the University of Texas. Thanks to a fellowship from the Center's Director, Stephen Enniss, I was able to travel to Austin and do this. While we never read each other's diaries and journals while he was alive, I felt that this was justified, as Aidan's diaries are largely records of fact, rather than private thoughts, and some have in fact been published in full.

At certain points, to protect the privacy of other people, names have been changed. The course of the twenty-nine years that we spent together has at some points been simplified or otherwise altered in the interests of readability. This is not the place to look for hard facts, but I hope it does justice to a man who enriched my life immeasurably.

Alannah Hopkin
Kinsale, Co. Cork
November 2020

PART I
The Thunderbolt
1986–88

Where to start? At the beginning, naturally, in 1986, with the thunderbolt – the *coup de foudre*.

I was thirty-seven, living near Kinsale, earning my living as a writer, sharing a house platonically with an amiable American piano technician and five cats. I had recently parted from Stan Gébler Davies, a fellow writer and journalist, originally the third member of our household, to whom I had, rather quaintly, been engaged. Somehow, in spite of the fireworks, we had remained good friends. I was happy with my work: having published two novels with Hamish Hamilton, I had recently signed a generous contract with another London publisher for a non-fiction book, and was supplementing my income by book reviewing. I enjoyed my independent life in the country, and did not miss London, where I had lived until 1982. I had a wide circle of friends in Kinsale, and several cousins, as it was my mother's home town. I also had a couple of boyfriends, both Dubliners, who visited occasionally. After some turbulent times with a married poet (English), who broke my heart, and then with my chaotic on and off 'fiancé' Stan, who had an increasingly serious drink problem, I was glad not to be in love, to be footloose and fancy free, captain of my own ship.

My friend Derek Mahon had been awaiting the arrival of 'Higgins', his friend the novelist Aidan Higgins, for some weeks. After many years out of Ireland – London, South

Africa, Berlin, Spain – Higgins was living in Wicklow. Seamus Heaney had told him that if he chose to return to live in Ireland he could be a founder member of an association of writers and artists called Aosdána, and the government would give him an annual income, a stipend known as the *Cnuas*, provided he dedicated himself full-time to writing. He was on the next plane, and after a quick visit to Dublin to seal the formalities and open a bank account, he headed for Wicklow, where his brother Colman was living.

Higgins was not happy in Wicklow. He was living three and a half miles from the town, and did not drive. His landlady, who had promised to be away most of the time, was instead in residence most of the time, making him feel awkward, crowded. He had no like-minded friends in the area apart from Colman and his wife Sylvia. Derek immediately solved his problem: he should move to Kinsale, a small town with twenty-three pubs and several resident writers, artists and other congenial, well-travelled companions. He gave Aidan my number, as someone who knew Kinsale well and might be able to help him find a cottage with a sea view at a reasonable rent. He rang me one evening. His voice was a pleasant surprise, what you would call an educated voice, more English than Irish, soft and gentle, a highbrow, ever so slightly superior voice, definitely the voice of a reader of *The Times Literary Supplement*, a man who would know a hawk from a handsaw.

Derek asked if I would help him to entertain Higgins, who was due any day. It was late October, but still dry and sunny. Kinsale looked gorgeous in its autumn colors, grey stone buildings against a blue sea. 'He's coming down by helicopter' was the latest news from Derek, followed by 'No sign of Higgins,' and days later, 'Still no sign of Higgins. And now they've cancelled the helicopter service.'

Another week went by. Stan rang to let me know he'd be back from London on Wednesday and invited me to dinner that night in the Captain's Cabin. Minutes later Derek rang. Higgins was arriving on Wednesday, could I join them for dinner? I apologised, and said I'd see them on Thursday. We agreed to meet as usual in the pool at Actons Hotel around six o'clock.

I remember having wet hair after my swim, and being too impatient to dry it, suddenly curious to see what this Higgins looked like. Suppose, I thought idly, he turns out to be someone significant in my life, and his first view of me is of an otter-like wet head. I dismissed this uncharacteristic romantic thought from my thoroughly rational mind and headed for the bar.

And there he was, in a wine-red wool sweater, medium height and build, long reddish-brown hair, granny glasses, slightly stooped, engaged in close conversation with an enormous bear of a man called Sven. Derek must have made the introductions, I do not remember, but I do remember Sven's handshake almost breaking my bones, while the touch of Higgins' hand was like velvet. Neither Sven nor Higgins was entirely sober. Sven was a sea captain, Higgins told me in that extraordinary voice, who had killed a man at sea in the course of his duties.

Derek had chosen to dine at the Shipwreck, a new place just behind the hotel. He did not drink, so Higgins and I quickly agreed on a bottle of Rioja. The pizzas were the worst any of us had ever tasted, tomato gloop topped by processed cheese and ham. Derek knew Aidan and I both had strong opinions about the writer Malcolm Lowry. I listened to Aidan telling me the theory that his Canadian friend had about Lowry – that in *Under the Volcano* he had completely misunderstood the political situation in Mexico –

and I liked the way he stood up for his friend's insight when I contradicted it. Lowry's fictional version of Mexican politics in 1937 is, in fact, totally accurate, and I had proved that in my MA dissertation. I liked the way he took me seriously, and didn't flirt. Higgins ordered another bottle of Rioja, at which point Derek politely said good night and left.

We first kissed in the car park, and Aidan's glasses fell apart. Mine often did the same, and I was able to retrieve the pieces and put them together. Aidan was struck dumb with admiration by my technical wizardry. I noticed that his eyes were hazel, exactly the same colour as mine. It was like looking into my own soul. The thunderbolt struck. I took his hand and led him to the car and drove the mile and a half home. We stayed in bed until the following afternoon, and did not see Derek again until the Saturday.

'A nice pair,' was his amused greeting, as we knocked contritely on his door. We had come to collect Aidan's things. We were moving in together.

It all sounds so simple – fall in love, move in together. I remember the first few weeks with Aidan as a time of euphoria, but that is not what I find in my journal from the time.

Thursday, 19 November 1986
All this emotion. I should be happy, should I not, and instead I feel like bursting into tears of rage – because the house is such a mess and stinks of cat piss, not to mention the cold – because I've lost a day and a half's work, and my whole hard-earned rhythm, because my concentration is absolutely shot – in short because I've met Aidan Higgins. An attack of cowardice perhaps, but also a long howl of 'Do I need this?' … Can I live without it?'

Certainly, get out quick is one reaction. The other is this terrible sense of things being pre-ordained, there is no escaping this fate ... ideally he should go back to Wicklow while I finish the St Patrick book and get on with quiet, sane living. But I'm sure he can be quiet too, once he gets off this bender, and he seems to respect my need to work. Hell! I haven't written a word of the book since last Friday. I have three weeks and a bit left before I go to visit my parents in London, thank God for London, it'll calm me down.

Aidan's Diary, 18 November 1986
Kinsale. Woke to raised voice, Mahon on phone to London. I left. Meet at Swedish Chef at midday. Pubs open at 10.30am. Into Armada. Mahon swimming at 7pm in new pool at hotel, meeting Alannah. Armada landlady English – London Irish. Child at bottle, I doze off before coal fire. Hours pass. Soup. Driven out by mixture of radio and TV news very loud. At hotel bar met Sven Jensen of Norwegian ship. Derek to pool – more bumping around than swimming due to smallness of pool he says. Bumperini. Sven a trout catcher. Watcher of fish. We are asked to move. Sitting when Derek returns. Then out of corner of eye, the femme fatale Alannah. Mixture of Hanne Vong and Nuala McAllister, old flames of yore. She had been swimming in the hotel swimming pool. I'd seen a photograph of her where she looked like an Italian lesbian (not that I have ever encountered one). The hair at the nape of her neck was damp; I thought she had something of the otter in her. She

had the delicateness of a cat, something quiet and feline, the voice pitched low, no discernible Irish accent, certainly not Cork. Skin. Drinking red wine. Survives bone-crushing handshake from sailor Sven who wants to be marine biologist. Shipwreck wine bar for 8pm. Follow Alannah. Place run by Englishman Jeff and Galway wife. Music off. A kitten and a red setter by turf fire. Derek departs as others arrive. Three Spaniards, Angel and amigos. Banter in Spanish with Alannah. Buying lobsters for export. We drink at counter, Cuban cigars, out to car, undecided. Lens falls from left eye. Alannah fixes. Stay until 3am. Back to her place. House shared with 4 or 5 smelly cats and American piano tuner. Encountered already in Swedish Chef. Undressed her, she me. Say 4.00am. Long dalliance. Darkness.

The next morning, driving into Kinsale, I had a very strong flash of intuition about Aidan, which led to a firm resolution. I was not going to let him, or the affair, become the most important thing in the world. He was a new part of my life, but all the rest was still there too. I was much stronger than before. I had learnt how to live in the present, enjoying what I do now, without worrying about the future, long or short term. I was getting to know him better, and liking what I saw. But if he were to disappear, I would not be distraught or feel let down. We were just testing, that's all, and very nice it was too. One step at a time.

A week later I moved out of the ramshackle house I'd been sharing with Tom Rourk and our five cats. It had started as a three-way rent share with Stan, whom we had evicted after a matter of days for being disruptive and uncooperative (less house-trained than the cats – they at least did not smoke slim panatellas in the bath). I felt shifty leaving Tom to pay the full rent after only a year, but it was a large house with four bedrooms, a short walk from the sea. I was sure he could find another housemate if he wanted to, and he was gracious about it. He kept my two cats for the time being, and I let him keep my furniture.

We were walking along Market Street a day later when it occurred to me to ask Aidan how old he was. I honestly had no idea. When he said 'Fifty-nine,' I thought at first that he was joking. 'Don't you mean forty-nine?' In fact, he could have passed for thirty-nine. But it didn't matter. If anybody had told me to think long and hard before getting involved with a man twenty-three years older than me, I would have told them to mind their own business. Aidan and I were obviously destined for each other, and what was a bit of an age difference in the face of true love? 'Love is not love which alters when it alteration finds…'

Aidan and I found a simple apartment in town, two rooms, kitchen and bathroom under the eaves of a tall narrow house known as the Dutch House because of its front gable. It was across the road and up a bit from a ruined stone tower house, Desmond Castle, also known as 'the French Prison' since fifty-four prisoners had perished in a fire there during the Napoleonic wars. The front windows of the Dutch House looked up a hill lined with pollarded plane trees leading to a church called the Friary, while the south-facing back window had a distant view of the harbour. A side window in the kitchen let in the western light. We told the landlord's wife, who was showing us around, that we'd take it. The rent was a very reasonable £340 a quarter, payable in advance – just under £25 a week. 'What sort of a deposit would you like?' Aidan asked. 'A fiver will do.'

I worked on my book, known at that time as *St Patrick and the Irish People*, at a table in the bedroom, where I could close the door on the rest of the apartment. I had a large electric typewriter that hummed loudly, and the closed door also suited Aidan, who liked his silence. The typescript was due in mid-March. I had finished most of the research, and was now writing it up. Aidan nicknamed me the Great Patrician Scholar. I do not usually answer to nicknames, but I couldn't resist that one.

Aidan gave notice to his landlady in Wicklow, and made a trip up by train to bring back his stuff. After more than two years living in Ireland, his 'stuff' consisted of two small suitcases of clothes, a manual typewriter and two cardboard boxes of books, notebooks and files. He travelled light, and left hardly a trace behind him. He was by nature tidy and unusually graceful, with small feet and hands. He moved around with the silence of a cat, and had the poise of a natural athlete. When young he had been a scratch golfer, and Captain of Cricket at Clongowes. After school he played for Phoenix, a well-respected Dublin cricket club. He often stood like a slip fielder, leaning slightly forward, hands cupped in anticipation. When he sat in an armchair with his legs crossed, reading, as he often did, he pointed the toe of his foot in an almost lady-like way. There is a portrait of his mother sitting reading outdoors in exactly the same posture.

In no time at all it seemed as if we had always lived together. There was an oddly continental feel to mornings in the Dutch House which began with a half-strangled cock crow that Aidan identified as a bantam cock. This was followed by tinny church bells and the cooing of pigeons. We enjoyed the ever-changing views over grey-slated rooftops to the harbour on one side, and the stone-built ruined castle keep on the other. We had to learn to negotiate the wooden roof beams, or eaves, one beside the cooker that made the kitchen feel like a ship's galley, and others in the bathroom and sitting room. On rainy nights we liked to listen to the rain drumming on the roof as we lay in bed, both on our backs, like effigies of a knight and his lady on a medieval tomb, holding hands.

We were both by nature quiet, prone to long silences, and we both liked to read with great intensity. Neither of us wanted a television, and Aidan persuaded me to do without my bedside radio. He had a small one for rugby matches, but it was not up to music. If I wanted to, I could listen to cassettes on headphones. Both accustomed to living alone, we continued to keep to our own daily routines. I liked to go from bed to desk, with only a shower and a quick stand-up breakfast in between. Aidan was usually up before me, and would often leave his socks soaking in the hand basin, as if he had forgotten that I would be following him through the bathroom. I liked his high level of personal hygiene, but was puzzled that he did not remember that I would be using the bathroom next. Reluctant to set a precedent by washing his socks myself, I called out 'Socks in the sink' and waved my toothbrush at him. (Start as you intend to go on.) I had to go through the same routine several times before he remembered not to wash his socks until I'd finished with the bathroom.

Apart from the socks in the sink, he was highly domesticated. He insisted on sharing the cooking, and made a meal from scratch at least twice a week. This would either be spaghetti bolognese, pork chops or roast pork fillet. In Wicklow Town, where he did his weekly shopping, the butcher would greet him with a cry of 'Here comes the pork fillet man.' Together we kept the Dutch House clean and tidy. I assumed his awareness of the chores that needed doing and his willingness to pull his weight were the result of his years with his first wife Jill, and their three sons. He had continued living in the family flat long after the marriage was over, partly to help with the children: three boys, the youngest of whom was five in 1970 when they moved back to London from Spain.

He liked my habit of picking wild flowers on our walks and arranging them in vases around the house. We bought some dark varnish to smarten up the furniture, and some adhesive red gingham to brighten up the kitchen table and disguise the fridge.

Once I got to the desk, I stayed there for most of the day, working on the book, venturing out around five to buy food and wine, and maybe dropping into a pub on the way home for a sociable drink. The last post left Kinsale at 5 p.m., and if I was sending off a review I would often run into a fellow-writer at the post office, and go for a drink. Besides Stan Gébler Davies, the poet Robert Nye reviewed for *The Times* of London and *The Scotsman*. An American, Howard R. Simpson, reviewed for the *Sacramento Bee*, Derek Mahon reviewed for the *Irish Times*, among others, while the poet Desmond O'Grady and his writer and poet girlfriend Ellen Beardsley were also regulars at the post office.

Aidan had his own routines, often disappearing in the morning, and not reappearing until evening. Sometimes he'd be walking, getting to know the new territory, and sometimes he'd be amusing himself in one or other of the town's twenty-three bars, or joining Derek, Tom Rourk and the blow-ins (as we call non-natives) who had coffee together in the Swedish Chef. There was Adrian Walker, an Englishman who had made a film about Antarctica that was narrated by Aidan's hero, Orson Welles; Rourk was a notorious raconteur and lover of the outdoors, whose home town was Thoreau's Concord; and Howard R. Simpson, a retired diplomat and military historian. The Spaniard, a spit and sawdust pub on the road to Summercove, was the lunchtime 'office' of Desmond O'Grady, a bibulous, well-travelled poet from Limerick.

Aidan had also made friends in a bar known as the Captain's Cabin, a late-night drinking den in a back street behind Actons Hotel, known, jokingly, as 'the bad part of town'. It was run by a colourful man orignally from Cornwall, Tom Menhennick, generally known as 'Mad Tom', and his beautiful but contrary wife, Miranda. It did not have a spirits licence or a beer licence, and was officially a restaurant. Mainly people bought wine by the bottle. Sometimes ribs or steaks were grilled over an open fire, but generally there was little food, and much drinking. Because it opened late, it was popular with staff from the town's restaurants. Kinsale had more than half a dozen bistro-style restaurants, mainly run by owner-chefs, unusual in 1987. So the crowd in the Cabin, as it was known, tended to be well-travelled and cosmopolitan, exactly to Aidan's taste. He enjoyed the banter between Tom and Miranda, June Pope's lovely smile, and discovered a couple who had lived for a while in Nerja, where Aidan had lived in the 1960s. There were the Spanish lads who were trading in lobsters, a Breton fisherman, Jean Marie, who both caught and exported shrimp, and the big blonde, Pat O'Mahony, a larger-than-life character who lived a couple of doors away in a house called Foxwell (try pronouncing that in a Northumberland accent). Pat, like many people who gravitated to Kinsale, was a versatile worker. She could run a restaurant as chef, manager, waitress or all three, and she was also a hairdresser. A plain-spoken woman, she told Aidan his beard needed trimming and his hair was a disgrace. She would come over the next day at five.

'How do you know where we live?'

'Everyone knows where you live, darling. The love-birds of the Dutch House.'

She took me on too. I've always hated going to the hairdresser, so it was a treat to have someone come to the house, much more fun than the salon ritual, and also much cheaper. Every six weeks or so we were 'tidied up' by Pat at home, with the bonus of a full briefing on the latest town gossip over a glass of wine.

Aidan had been working on a new radio play, *Assassin*, based on the assassination of Archduke Franz Ferdinand in 1914 by Gavrilo Princip. Now the Abbey Theatre was showing interest in a stage version of the script, and he was corresponding with the Abbey's director, Vincent Dowling, about this. He was also tinkering with a couple of stories.

There was a coin-operated payphone in the hall of the Dutch House which we shared with the occupants of the two other apartments – Stan Gébler Davies on the ground floor (Kinsale is a very small town) and a musician called Frank Buckley in the middle. Frank made wine, and a great waft of fermenting matter belched out of his front door whenever it opened. He had a piano in his apartment, and gave private lessons to beautiful young singers. On weekdays he taught music in the local school, and on Saturdays he conducted the music for weddings and on Sundays the church choir. No wonder he was usually seen running, briefcase in one hand, car keys in the other, coat tails flying out behind him as he made his way from one engagement to the other. Aidan noted in his diary at this time, 'Buck leaping downstairs humming "Where the mountains of Mourne sweep down to the sea" after thirty minutes piano of same.' Frank also composed, and there was always a pile of hand-written music manuscripts behind the front door, as if Haydn had been working on his symphony.

On Wednesday 3 December, soon after moving into the Dutch House, we began a Scrabble tournament. We played every evening around six, and Aidan kept a record in hardback school nature notebooks of every word played in every game. He won the first one by a respectable thirty-one points. We were well-matched, but I had the edge on him for vocabulary due to my interest in gardening, cooking, sailing and horses. We were competitive, but agreed not to become Scrabble bores and memorise lists of unusual two-letter words. Rather than consulting the official Scrabble-players' dictionary, Chambers, our authority was my two-volume Shorter Oxford Dictionary, because it was what we had in the house. If a word was not found in the Shorter Oxford, it was not allowed. The game was usually over in an hour, but sometimes it could last longer, which tried my patience. Before meeting Aidan this time of day had been reading time. But Aidan obviously relished the ongoing Scrabble rivalry, so it seemed churlish to refuse. It was also a good way of continuing to get to know each other, as we competed for word-domination. What began as a casual pastime turned into a serious tournament, and Scrabble-time, 6 p.m., became a fixture in our daily routine.

Within days of starting the Scrabble tournament, we both had Scrabble nicknames. He had trounced me in a game by putting 'squid' on a double-letter score with the Q on a triple-letter tile, and I took to calling him 'Squid'. I liked the familiarity of it, the way it made him mine. 'Aidan' in contrast seemed formal and remote, a little like his voice, someone older and perhaps wiser, whereas Squid cut him down to size, made him seem human.

I acquired the nickname Zinnia in a similar way, putting the letter Z on a triple-letter tile, and the whole thing on a double-word score. But Aidan challenged the validity of zinnia, claiming that it was a proper noun with a capital Z and therefore not allowed in Scrabble. It's a flower, I protested, it's the national flower of Mexico and it doesn't have a capital letter, but still we had to look it up. If it was in the OED I would win tonight's game of Scrabble.

I checked the OED: There it was: zinnia! I had won. He gave me many nicknames, but the only one that stuck was Zinnia, often shortened to Zin.

Aidan noted in his diary in December 1986: 'They played the word-game called Scrabble. She put down Zinnia, he put down Squid. She put down quim, he put down swived. She: obligato, he: muzzle, she: atremble, he: susceptible, she: warm, he: somnolent.'

Early on Aidan and I had agreed not to use the 'L' word. We seldom referred to it, and when we did we preferred to use the 'A' word: *amor*. We were so obviously smitten with each other, there was really no need to break the spell by putting such strong feelings into the usual banal words – clichés, words already used with other people, scarred by past betrayals, words that for all their oath-like qualities do not belong to the moment which needs no saying. Words give no protection against the future, reducing the sublime to time-worn old phrases. Better the purity of silence. Show, don't tell became the rule. Somehow it made everything more exciting, two almost-silent people taking each other totally on trust. We kept terrible hours, because we could, and often gave more importance to making love than to turning up at the desk. There were always weekends on which to catch up. We talked a lot in bed, probably more than anywhere else. There's a terrible fear when something starts off so well, that it can only go downhill. But not us: AH + AH. Or AH^2.

Obviously destined for each other.

Talking in Bed

Early one morning, I named my ex-love, the last one that mattered. The English poet. Four years ago. Before Stan. I said he had pursued me with every trick in the book.

'Every trick in the book?' asked Aidan, solemnly. 'I didn't know there were such books. Books containing lists of tricks?' It was the start of a long-running campaign to encourage me to stop using clichés, and to choose my words with more precision.

Aidan had named three other women. Three in the course of so many years. Elin, Nanna, Anastasia.

'In retrospect, perhaps I'm susceptible. But nothing like this.'

Rain coming down sideways outside, gale howling for the duration. Roof threatening to lift off with the force of the storm. Never had there been anything like this.

He asked me to keep telling him that I was happy with him. *Lo soy. Estoy muy contenta.* He liked me to talk simple Spanish, and seemed to understand it. He had what he called 'bar Spanish'. His favourite word was '*Depende*', which cleverly gave the impression he knew a lot more Spanish than he actually did.

But 'Roll with the punches,' he kept saying.

(Will that help when they come, as come they must?)

He was worried about being so much older than me, but while I saw it as a long-term worry, and therefore not important at the moment, he saw it as an immediate problem. He said that I reminded him of a lot of people, meaning other women; did he remind me of anyone? Yes, I said firmly, with no hint that I would add anything to it. I think that he was nonplussed. Like the man who had used every trick in the book, Aidan had a full beard, glasses, dark brown hair and was a brilliant talker who made me laugh. Aidan was older than his predecessor, and his eyes were not as mad, but there was a definite resemblance, extending even to corduroy trousers, suede shoes and a Donegal tweed jacket.

Sometimes being of a certain age, thirty-seven, is no help at all. Falling in love was almost as incapacitating as it had been at nineteen, except that this time round you know it can suddenly turn bad, you learn to anticipate it, even in the midst of great happiness. As a prophylactic against dullness, I was determined not to become too close, not to share everything with the new beloved, to keep some secrets. Co-dependency is the enemy of romance, that much I knew. I told him I would never read his letters or his diaries, unless he wanted me to. He agreed to respect my written privacy too, and I asked him to extend it to all work-in-progress. I have a horror of people reading what I've written before it is properly finished.

*

I was hoping Aidan would like my work. That was the main thing. But when I took another look at my first novel, *A Joke Goes a Long Way in the Country*, I discovered that on the very first page the narrator has abandoned a book by Aidan Higgins on the floor beside her sofa: 'The floor around her was littered with discarded books, Seamus Heaney, J. G. Farrell, Aidan Higgins, Bernard MacLaverty, Desmond Hogan, Julia O'Faolain, Jennifer Johnston, most of them resting face down, open at the page where she'd lost interest. She preferred to look at the burning turf and listen to the rain.'

I wrote in my journal at the time: 'My fear is that all of a sudden he will hurt me, turn on me, not abandoning me like X did, but the same level of hurt in the end. Let's face it (oh, horrible expression), I'm afraid he might dislike my writing, or refuse to take it seriously. Question is, do we get it over today, or do I let it drift on?'

Next day's entry: 'Aidan read *A Joke* – as far as page 67. Verdict: "Not interesting."'

It was a cold verdict, it hurt, but I tried to preserve a professional façade. It was, truth to tell, very much a first novel, self-obsessed and rather pleased with its own effects. I had written it purely for myself, to see if I could, and to keep me busy on quiet weekends when I was living alone in Soho. What he said when pressed was 'too many *muletas*, not enough *piquetes*', i.e. too much cape work, and not enough thrusts to the core – the place where it hurts. I fought back of course, while half-agreeing. He also said that Alex (the main character) is not me. He said I am probably too nice to write a good novel – which I thought (a) showed how little he knew me and (b) was a very strange notion. I said, 'I can be very nasty on occasion,' and he said, 'That's the spirit,' which I found patronising. He then added that I did not need praise and flattery – I had had too much of that. I needed to be told what's wrong with my writing, not what is good.

Then he told me an anecdote from Lauren Bacall's autobiography about a Broadway producer who always sent away impossibly bad playwrights loaded with praise – the script is wonderful, perfect, you'll be hearing from me, etc., while those that he liked, who had promise, he utterly tore apart and sent off to rewrite, because he knew that would get good results.

He should have told me that story first. It would have hurt less.

As I thought it over, I could see that from my supporters all I ever got was praise, which really didn't help. In fact in less than ten minutes Aidan had given me more constructive advice about my work than I had ever had so far.

Is it any wonder that I was falling in love with him?

One evening, after Scrabble, I was doodling with pen and paper, and discovered that Aidan's name contained a perfect anagram: Diana Gishing. He was delighted with it, and immediately characterised her as a fastidious retired headmistress. He often used the name to sign letters to the editor, of a complaining nature. This appeared in Michael Viney's column in the *Irish Times* on 2 June 1990:

> *An Eye on Nature*
> *How many bluebottles will breed out of one dead mouse? The dead mouse cannot be reached inside the wall and bluebottles emerge at an average rate of, say, 80 a day, now a week old. How many maggots from the corpse and what rate of reproduction, and when does it end?*
> *Diana Gishing, Kinsale, Co Cork*

Michael Viney replied:

> *Very soon now. The eggs laid by one bluebottle vary according to food supply, but often weigh more in total than she does. They hatch within a day or two, the maggots grow a few days more, and the pupa releases the full-grown fly after that. Each female bluebottle now buzzing at the window will lead to several more generations during the summer.*

The best I could come up with for Derek Mahon was a Dutchman, Mark de Hoen, not nearly as successful. Derek took to addressing the postcards he and Aidan often wrote to each other to Diana Gishing, and they were duly delivered.

In spite of dropping his name on the first page of my first novel, I had not even read *Langrishe, Go Down* (1966), Aidan's best-known novel, before I met him. I had read a lukewarm review of *Balcony of Europe* (1972) many years ago, which classified it as a failure, opining that Aidan had spent too much time drinking in the bars of southern Spain, and not enough time editing his novel, which was far too long, and unfocused. As a result I had not felt the need to seek it out. Nor had I read his subseqent novel, *Scenes from A Receding Past* (1978), nor his most recent one, *Bornholm Night-Ferry* (1983).

Aidan had an unusual publishing history. He was first published by John Calder, to whom he had been recommended by Samuel Beckett. When lack of money forced his parents to sell the family home, Springfield, a Georgian house with stables and seventy-two acres in Celbridge, County Kildare, they had moved to a modest suburban house on the Burnaby Estate in Greystones, an upmarket estate popular with affluent Protestants in a seaside village on the railway line between Wicklow and Dublin. The family next door were typical – Gerald Beckett was a doctor working as Medical Officer for Wicklow County Council, a post based in Rathdrum, in the far south of the county. His wife, Peggy, a native of Sandymount in Dublin, wanted to live as close to the city as possible, and as a compromise they chose Greystones. Their son John and Aidan were the same age, and became good friends. John (later a musican and composer) was as passionate about music as Aidan was about reading and writing. John loaned Aidan four books; three of them made no impression at all on him, but the fourth, John's cousin Samuel Beckett's novel *Murphy*, 'raised the hair on his head ... It was the business'.[1] When John's mother Peggy found out how much he liked the book, she sent him to visit the composer Walter Beckett in Donnybrook, who gave him a copy of *More Pricks than Kicks*, discreetly wrapped in brown paper. Aidan wrote an admiring letter to Samuel, but John told him there was no use posting it, as Sam never answered letters. This time he did, but alas, Aidan was unable to decipher the handwriting. But Peggy managed to make it out: 'Despair young, and never look back.' It was the start of a long friendship, much of it conducted by letter. When Aidan's first collection of stories was ready, Samuel Beckett recommended it to his publisher, John Calder, who immediately took it on.

During my last years in London I had been friendly with Gary Pulsifer, a young American, who was running John Calder's office in Brewer Street. When it was closing time at the French pub, Gary and I and a few others would sometimes go back to the office with more wine to continue our conversation. I'd end up browsing the bookshelves, but I don't remember ever seeing Aidan's books there: Samuel Beckett, yes, and John Calder's excellent book on his work; Raymond Queneau, Nathalie Sarraute, Alain Robbe-Grillet yes, but Aidan Higgins? *Images of Africa*? *Felo de Se*? *Langrishe, Go Down*? *Balcony of Europe*? *Scenes from a Receding Past*? No. I can't say I noticed his name or his books.

When Aidan came back from Wicklow with his stuff he gave me a copy of *Langrishe, Go Down*, which would have to wait until I had more reading time, and a much shorter one, *Images of Africa*, a book of travel writing that appeared in John Calder's Signature series of shorter works. My copy of *Images of Africa* has a hand-written dedication, For Zinnia, then the line drawing of a wine glass filled with a blob of red ink, which always accompanied his signature among family and friends, and the word 'Aidan'.

I far preferred this slim volume to what I had glimpsed of *Langrishe*. I immediately loved the spareness and precision of his prose, and the fact that he had written a very short book about three years spent touring Africa with a puppet company, not the long boring tome that most aspiring writers would have produced. This is what Calder wrote for the dust jacket of *Images*: 'A writer's private thoughts – which are at once perceptive, detached and compassionate – are set down here at random to make a unique documentary. Individuals, sketched in the briefest of phrases, explode into life. A diary this may be but it has all the ingredients of a stylistic masterpiece.'

The epigraph is that chilling paragraph from *Robinson Crusoe* in which Friday and Robin discover the natives on the beach 'eating the flesh of one of their prisoners', while another bearded white man lies nearby, trussed up, waiting his turn. I read the opening paragraph of Aidan's text, a chapter called 'The Voyage':

The plunge over the equator. Flying fish sink, porpoises rise, and evening after evening the sun goes down in formations of cloud, furnace-like, dramatic as anything in Doré's illustrations to Dante. The approaches to a new continent. Such lovely leewardings! They must lead somewhere.

The hairs on the back of my neck rose up. For once a book lived up to its publisher's claims. Now I understood why people praised Higgins as a stylist. Here indeed was a *maestro*. I noted in my journal 'Read *Images of Africa* on Friday evening, a most beautiful book. Such economy, such strength, so much left out. So many beautiful scenes. For once the blurb got it right, "perceptive, detached and compassionate".'

In fact, this extraordinary little book only came out because there was a printer's strike in between the appearance of Aidan's first collection of stories, *Felo de Se*, and *Langrishe, Go Down*, which created a two-year gap. As his publisher, Calder wanted to keep Aidan's name before the reading public, so he asked if he had anything that would sit well among the slim volumes of the Signatures series. Aidan dug up an old notebook which became, pretty much word for word, *Images of Africa*.

Alannah's Diary, 11 December 1986
Aidan read *The Out-haul* in one sitting, and talked to me at length about it yesterday. It was a hot-whiskey day, dark, with a high wind, so we walked to the Dock for three of them. It's a good bar in winter, almost empty except for a few silent locals, the dark green Godin stove throwing out heat. He says I must change my angle of attack, watch the adverbs and adjectives – they are too cosying. He recommends using simple declarative sentences, paying more attention to the olfactory sense – only one smell mentioned in the whole novel, the smell while untacking the horses. Pay more attention to all the senses, write with all of them. Which means taking more notes. It was all said in the kindest

possible way, he believes that I can write ten times better. He praised my poems, especially 'The Gift of Woodcock': they showed what I could do; the novel did not.

It would have been good if he had liked it, I cannot deny I am disappointed. And I am not quite sure he was reading it with an open mind, open to what I was doing in the novel, not what he thought I should be doing … But look, it's only my second novel, he's been writing so much longer than me. The age gap is not about him being 23 years older than me, it is that he has been working as a writer for 23 years longer than I have: I am still a novice by comparison. He is the best, and I must not get discouraged by comparisons.

There was much talk in the Dock about 'our house'. The one we are going to buy together. It is so long since I've used the first person plural. There has been too much 'I' and not enough 'we' in my life over the past ten years. We want a big Godin stove which also heats radiators, and a small wood burning stove in each work room. We will spend January and February of each year in Spain. He is very confident of his ability to earn more money. He has a play, 'Assassin', which is being considered by the Abbey, but could still be produced as a radio play as well. He has a travel script that might make a film for Lindsay Anderson, and two collections coming out in London next year, travel writing and stories. 'Keep sending it out in all media,' he says, 'And we shall have a house.'

How wonderful to know someone who is not broke!

Some three weeks after meeting Aidan, I went on a long-promised trip to London to spend Christmas with my parents. I would have preferred to stay with him in our new home, but I had promised to visit my parents, and could not let my increasingly frail mother down. Also I needed to do some work on St Patrick in the London Library. I took the copy of *Langrishe, Go Down* he had given me to London, and I read it in in my parents' flat, with its familiar view across the River Thames to Battersea Park. It was a way of staying close to Aidan, though physically absent.

While it certainly had some extraordinarily vivid passages of writing – the masterly opening sequence of a queasy Helen on the Celbridge bus at twilight, for example – it was too traditional for my taste, with its intricately worked sentences, and leisurely narrative pace. I preferred writing that came fresh off the page, as if new-minted, writing that had no respect for literary conventions nor highbrow references – like the writing I had found in *Images of Africa*.

I remember being in a state of total euphoria for the whole of that trip, and I probably spoke of nothing but Aidan. When my father heard soon after I arrived that I had 'met someone' he immediately opened a bottle of champagne. I had Bizet's *Carmen*, the full opera, on cassettes that I played constantly at full volume through the headphones of my Walkman:

L'amour est enfant de Bohème,
il n'a jamais jamais connu de loi,
si tu ne m'aime pas je t'aime,
et si je t'aime PRENDS GARDE À TOI....

In the London Library that December, while taking a break from Patrician studies, I found a well-worn copy

of *Bornholm Night-Ferry*, an epistolary novel published
in 1983 based on Aidan's affair with a Danish poet, and I
was immediately enthralled. This was more like my sort
of thing, a bold experiment in language, that was also a
compelling love story. It was a bizarre experience, to be
reading this vivid account of the man I had just fallen in
love with, falling deeply in love with someone else. But the
writing was so wonderful, so strong and so strange that
nothing else mattered. The voice in the letters, written by
an Irish novelist called Fitz, was essentially his own voice;
there were none of the convoluted literary sentences that
had spoilt *Langrishe* for me. And I could cope with my
conflicted feelings, the natural inclination to jealousy when
reading about someone else who had been in his life before
me, because I knew that it did not matter any more: it
was he and I who mattered now. We had agreed from the
start that, meeting at the age we did, there was no point
in retrospective jealousy. We had both lived lives before we
met, been in love, married, had affairs, and in his case three
children. Now we were starting again, starting anew.

Aidan's Diary, 23 December 1986
Taken up with Anglo Irish lady Alannah Lee Hopkin
born in Singapore, her Dad a doctor at the Fall,
Changi internee. Wedded to Mexican photographer
who wants to be architect. Lived in Mexico City for
two years before marriage broke up, speaks fluent
Spanish, good (fair) French. Published two novels,
not proof against the mildew of the stock phrase.
37 years. An evening swimmer. Never (rarely)
lachrymose. In appearance: a mixture of Oja Kodar
and Tusse Silberg. Wears contact lenses. That look
you get from myopic eyes.

I rang the Dutch House at lunchtime on Christmas Day, wishing I could be in Kinsale instead of cooking a turkey in my parents' flat in Chelsea. Aidan answered. He and Derek had been for a walk on a cold, sunny day, and now they were having lunch together. What were they eating?

'A fry.'

★

I got back from London on 3 January 1987. It was bitterly cold, but I insisted on a walk out to the lighthouse on the Old Head of Kinsale. This was a popular walk along the rough grass of an exposed headland, past a ruined de Courcey castle across increasingly high ground, to a narrow promontory, lashed by crosswinds, usually blowing west to east. At some points the grass, ungrazed for many years, was so springy that you could bounce on it, like a trampoline. If the wind was strong enough, you could lean into it with your full weight, and remain upright. The gulls and cliffs of the Old Head reminded Aidan of the Aran Isles, while the sea on either side recalled the long voyage out to South Africa on an ocean liner, sixteen days at sea, and the boredom of shipboard life. The walk to the lighthouse was a ritual, to be performed as soon as possible after getting home from London, to blow away the bad city air and ground myself again.

Aidan often told me about the long, Benzedrine-and-wine-fuelled walks he used to take in Andalucía, in the hills around Nerja with his friend Harry Calnek, a Canadian journalist, and other pals. He had a habit of talking about his friends, usually by surname only, as if I knew who they were, and I often had to ask for explanations – remind me again who Calnek is. Poole – was he the one your wife had an affair with? Who is Donal? John Deck? There was never any mention of a woman on these walks, and I suspected he thought women would not be up to it. I became competitive in my walking, and would never admit to being tired or wanting to turn back, to show that I was as good a walker as any man.

So I would not admit to finding the Old Head walk unusually cold and windy on that day, though perhaps it was. Aidan came down with a heavy cold that laid him low for 'a fortnight' as he always said, an approximation, I soon discovered, indicating a long period of time, not specifically 'two weeks'. He had no hesitation in blaming the Old Head walk for his illness. 'Then why haven't I got a cold?' I asked, and he had no answer. It was the start of his wariness of taking walks with me, and I have to admit the walks were sometimes challenging. But he was a strong, healthy man, surely he was well up to anything I could do?

After Christmas we continued to rent the Dutch House but moved for the rest of the winter, at my parents' suggestion, to my mother's house, their holiday home, beside the sea in a village a mile down the coast from Kinsale called Summercove. The house was on three floors, and had four bedrooms, which allowed us to spread ourselves out and have a work room each. In return, we paid the heating bills, and kept an eye out for storm damage. In the summer, or whenever my parents or other family members would want to use the house, we would retreat with our books and papers to the Dutch House.

I had lived in the Summercove house alone for my first two years in Ireland while I found out whether it was possible to earn a living so far from London. It was just across the road from the sea, looking out on a small stone-built pier, and right next door to a pub, the Bulman. The landlord was a keen card player, and there were regular good-natured games of poker, ten pence in and half the pot maximum bet, among a small group of locals. Aidan was immediately accepted, and spent many daytime hours in there, taking the notes that he used eventually in his Battle of Kinsale story, 'Sodden Fields'.[2] Meanwhile, I was working steadily towards the 17 March deadline of the St Patrick book. By then I had to have a good first draft in the post to London in order to get my next slice of the advance.

Summercove was my territory. I had spent most of my childhood summers in the village, where my mother had gone to school and lived until 1932, when she went to study nursing in London, where she met my English father. I knew everybody in Summercove, and their story. Many of the characters in my second novel, *The Out-haul*, were composites based on originals I'd met in the Bulman. For some time now I had been working on a short story set in the pub, eventually published as 'An Explanation of the Tides'.[3] Our neighbours Joe and Fred Revatto, an idle younger man named Thomas O'Leary, Helen Fair the bar person, and Willie O'Brien the landlord, were all recreated on the page by Aidan in 'Sodden Fields'. We were there too in 'Sodden Fields', Peter Storm (named for the make of Aidan's oilskin jacket) and his dark-haired fancy woman, striding out in all weathers to take the air after a long day at the desk. Or not at the desk. Thomas became Tomás following an impassioned conversation about the Irish language, and then 'the Great O'Leary', which was somehow related to Yeats's poem 'September 1913', with its famous line 'Romantic Ireland's dead and gone, / It's with O'Leary in the grave'.

O'Leary had long blond hair down his back, and was missing most of his front teeth. He had moved out of the family home and was living in a caravan up the lane behind the pub. He had lived and worked in Israel and Iceland and on off-shore oil rigs, and was still only thirty-two. He was currently living off a generous insurance payment from the oil rig for a broken thumb. The older men who came to the Bulman an hour or so before closing time for their couple of pints disliked O'Leary for his bad language, and if he was still in the pub, they always sat as far away from him as they could. His language was indeed blue, but he had a sharp wit, read the *Irish Examiner* daily from cover to cover, did the cryptic crossword, and played a good game of poker. Aidan and he enjoyed a kind of verbal jousting, and there was often loud laughter from their corner of the bar.

★

Even though we were living together, we still had separate lives, and did not do everything as a couple. I did not want one of those symbiotic relationships where you live in each other's pockets and become so close that romance goes out the window. A little difference and a few mysteries are good. As already agreed, we did not read each other's mail, nor necessarily share whatever news the post had brought – and this was a time when all serious news arrived in a letter or on a postcard. I did not read his diary, ever, or his notebooks, and in theory he did not read mine. Nor did we read each other our work-in-progress, ever. The very idea made me feel queasy.

One of the things I most liked about Aidan was that he showed no signs of expecting me to change my way of life to suit him, nor did he impose his company on me all the time. We were both quiet, not inclined to chat. Though when out walking, I had learned to exchange casual small talk, Irish-style, and had perfected a technique of shouting 'Shocking!' or 'Diabolical', 'Fine day!' or 'Great to see the sun!' to people as I walked past, without actually stopping to chat. Aidan had a reputation in Dublin literary circles for being difficult and contrary, partly because he simply did not do small talk. I had been so silent as a child that for many years my mother feared I was a bit strange.

True to my determination not to change my way of life just because I had a new partner, I continued to stay out late at night when I felt like it, usually with Stan and other friends, going back to his flat which had a TV and a stereo (unlike ours) after pub-closing time. If I woke Aidan by accident when I came home, he could be tetchy, and we might have a minor spat (as he called it), but we always made it up quickly, and we never let the sun go down on a disagreement. He and Stan were pals at this time, having long conversations in the afternoons in Stan's local, the Armada. Occasionally they stayed up all night together, playing chess and smoking slim panatellas. We could always tell when Stan was back from London by the smell of these permeating the hall outside his door. Following an occasion on which Stan gave Aidan a detailed explanation of his Bohemian ancestry on the Gébler side, Aidan nicknamed him 'the Baron', and never called him anything else.

I was not back from London for long when I ran into Tom Rourk, my former housemate, as I was leaving the post office one evening. Unusually, we went for a drink. I did not dislike Tom, but I'd had more than enough of his company during the year and a bit we'd shared a house, and felt no need to socialise with him. He was prone to leisurely anecdotes, for which I had little patience. He seemed to have some exciting news, a smug air of 'I know something that you don't know' about him.

This time the anecdote concerned a conversation between Aidan and Derek while enjoying a roast chicken that Tom had cooked for them while I was away. Derek had said something complimentary about *The Out-haul*, and Aidan had countered it with a total demolition of the novel. It was a terrible piece of writing. He picked up the book and opened it apparently at random. He read out a sentence, part of a description of a quiet Christmas Day in BallyC (the fictional village in which the novel is set): 'Small, thoughtful presents were exchanged.' He then lectured the company on why that was an atrocious piece of writing – the use of the passive voice, the lack of specificity, the cosy narrative tone. According to him, the novel was a terrible piece of work, and I was a terrible writer.

I was aware of Tom studying me closely to see how I was taking his piece of news. I was damned if I was going to let him see how much it angered me. 'Well, everyone's entitled to their opinon,' I said, draining my drink in order to make a quick getaway. It was not as if I was going to dissolve in tears; I didn't do that sort of thing. I was angry rather than hurt: Aidan could say what he liked about my work to me in person, one to one, and I could take it. I could take anything that would help me to write better, that was the one thing in life that interested me. But I could not take someone who apparently loved me, going around and poisoning one of the few admirers of my work against it.

Or could I? Was I going to challenge Aidan about his disloyalty or not? The obvious next move was to have no more to do with him, to walk away and renounce his company for ever. But did I have the nerve, did I have the steel for that?

I had left a promising freelance career in London and moved to Ireland in 1982 in the belief that I would be living mainly on what I earned from writing fiction. When it turned out that Hamish Hamilton were not going to commission a third novel, given the disappointing sales of the first two, I reverted to earning a living from journalism. Seán Lucy, professor of English at University College Cork, kindly gave me some hours tutoring first-year students, in the belief that contact with a working writer would be good for them. In whatever spare time I had, I worked on a novel set in eighteenth-century west Cork.

I had been finding it very hard to survive on what I earned from tutoring at UCC, plus reviewing and writing occasional travel or arts features. Life was fun and full of variety, but there was just not enough money coming in, even though I was writing for the *Financial Times*, the *Irish Times*, *The Guardian*, the *Mail on Sunday*'s magazine *You* and *Time Out*, as well as updating Fodor's Guide to Ireland every year. If I could qualify for membership of Aosdána, like Aidan and Derek, I would be eligible for the same basic income that they both lived on, the *Cnuas*. It seemed like a logical next move. Ernest Gébler, Stan's uncle, a successful commercial novelist, who had been mentoring me since I moved to Ireland, proposed me, and I was seconded by Derek Mahon, one of a new wave of Northern Irish poets including Seamus Heaney and Michael Longley. It seemed a good combination, the older prose writer and the younger poet. I would be coming up for election at the next annual general meeting.

Several times after first moving to Ireland I was reduced to returning to London for a few weeks, and staying with my ever-patient parents in order to work in-house at my old job with the listings magazine, *Time Out*, and save some money. I hit a particularly low point over Christmas 1985 and was persuaded to change agent, from the excellent but rather staid literary agency, A. D. Peters (chosen because the company had been Malcolm Lowry's agent), to the more commercial Reg Davis-Poynter. Within weeks, Reg had secured me a low five-figure advance from Grafton Books for a book about St Patrick. My money worries were over, for a year or so at least.

Aidan had enough to live on simply from his *Cnuas*, but the problem was, we were not living simply. I paid my share of the bills, and we kept separate bank accounts. But he was not as well off as he thought he was. I soon realised that the illusion that I had met someone who was not broke was just that. Too much money was being spent in bars, on bottles of good Rioja, and restaurant meals. One of Aidan's favourite sayings was 'May the giving hand never waver,' and certainly his never did. He had an overdraft in Wicklow, due to the punitive sum of money demanded from him by his landlady for repairs and cleaning when he left the cottage, and in no time at all, he also had an overdraft in Kinsale. He was still writing radio plays, and offering pieces of prose to the *London Magazine* and other literary reviews, but he seldom earned any money. Realising how much Derek, Stan and I were earning from reviewing, he started to introduce himself to the editors of national dailies and weekly magazines with the hope of picking up regular work. At that time he was trying to locate two typescripts he had lost track of in London and also chasing a backlog of royalties due to him from his other publisher, John Calder, who still had several books of his in print. After hearing his sorry tale one night in the Armada, Stan and I suggested that he ask our agent, Reg Davis-Poynter, to sort out the mess. Reg, who was familiar with Aidan's work, willingly took him on, agreeing to find him a new publisher, possibly Liz Calder (no relation) at Bloomsbury, which was just starting up.

Aidan read constantly, often rereading books that he liked – Karen Blixen's *Out of Africa* had come down from Wicklow with him, and also the stories of John Cheever and V. S. Pritchett, a couple of novels by Saul Bellow, Paul Theroux's travel writing and early novels. Soon after we met he gave me a copy of *Nightwood* by Djuna Barnes, a work that he greatly esteemed. At one time he had been able to recite by heart the opening three or four pages, and could still manage the long opening sentence. But he told me he had wrung *Nightwood* dry, read it too often, and it no longer gave him the pleasure it once had. He had done the same, he said, when he was younger, with Joyce's *A Portrait of the Artist as a Young Man*. The first time he read it, he imagined it had been written specifically for him, so he read it over and over again. But alas, *Nightwood*'s high baroque style did not appeal to me, and while acknowledging that it was a remarkable book, I could not pretend that I loved it as he did. One of the few writers we had both read and liked was Cyril Connolly. New editions of *Enemies of Promise* and *The Unquiet Grave* were soon up on the bookshelf to be reread and savoured afresh, the best bits read out loud: '…the true function of a writer is to produce a masterpiece, and no other task is of any consequence.' There was one thing at least that we could agree on.

Once settled in Kinsale, besides making notes for 'Sodden Fields', Aidan set to work rewriting and expanding 'The Bird I Fancied', a story about Mary, the woman who had been his girlfriend in London intermittently for around two years. The last week he spent in London, the start of a bender that would lead him, ten days later, via Cootehill, Cavan, Dublin and Greystones, to Kinsale, had made him realise that, much as he liked Mary's high spirits, her chaotic lifestyle, which included a large and possessive biker husband, made her an impossible long-term companion. Having met someone else, and moved to Kinsale, he could now look back at their long relationship from a new point of view. He was also reappraising himself in advance of his sixtieth birthday, which was coming up on 3 March.

As well as tapping away at his manual typewriter, Aidan would spend hours with his notebook, a hard-backed A4-sized one, in which he jotted down anything that caught his interest in his reading, as well as phrases and stories that he came across while eavesdropping in daytime bars or talking to locals, including his pal Tomás. Dole day was always a good source of stories from the many locals who had served in the merchant navy, and celebrated dole day by having a few pints. One afternoon he came back amazed to recount that he had been drinking with a man who had been the purser of the *Warwick Castle* on the same voyage on which he and Jill had sailed back from South Africa. The ship had left East London on 28 July 1960, and called at Port Elizabeth, Capetown, St Helena, the Canary Islands and Tilbury Docks. There had been a burial at sea off St Helena on that voyage, an unusual event marked by a simple ceremony presided over by the captain, which they both remembered. This odd coincidence confirmed Aidan's feeling that Kinsale was the right place for him to live. He was far more superstitious than I was, and had a hippie-like belief in star signs (he was proud of being a Pisces, the water sign). He played this down when I, being sceptical of astrology, was around, but shared it enthusiastically with fellow believers.

*

In January I drove us to the bus station to collect Carl and Carlota, unsure who I was about to meet. Aidan spoke of his eldest son as if he were a law unto himself, but also with warm affection. He liked to say that Carl should have been born in another century: he was like a character out of *The Three Musketeers* in his optimism and enthusiasm.

Through one of those flukes that often seem to happen when you fall in love, Aidan's eldest son Carl was married to a Mexican, Carlota, and I had spent time in Mexico, where my sister lives, and been briefly married to a Mexican. Carl worked as a film projectionist near his home in Muswell Hill. They had met in London, where Carlota had gone to improve her English. They were about to return to Mexico City, where Carlota's father had promised to set Carl up in business. Before they left, they wanted to come to Ireland to say goodbye to Aidan.

Aidan's sons had been brought up to call their parents Jill and Aidan. The two eldest, Carl and Julien, had grown up mainly in Spain, and were fluent in Spanish. Carl was almost exactly ten years younger than me. The family moved back to London in 1970 chiefly for the sake of the boys' education. Through a friend, Jill had achieved the impossible, and managed to rent a spacious unfurnished flat on the fifth floor of a mansion block on Muswell Hill Broadway, with a panoramic view over the City of London. Carl, who was then eleven, had been to school mainly in Spanish, and for a year in German, but never in English, which he did not speak as well as he spoke Spanish. He could hardly write at all in English, laboriously spelling the words out phonetically, as he had learnt to do in Spanish. He was thought to be severely dyslexic. Julien, two years younger, a quiet, thoughtful boy, also struggled with the discipline of formal education, but had no trouble reading or writing. Both were talented artists. Elwin, a cheerful, out-going character, aged five on their arrival at Muswell

Hill, settled in immediately, acquired a wide circle of friends and did reasonably well at school.

There had been some confusion about the bus schedule and the pair had been sitting arm in arm in the bus station in Cork for an hour by the time we got there. But they were not at all cast down, and Carl's obvious pleasure at being reunited with Aidan was good to see. It was high tide on the wooded creek beside the road approaching Kinsale, and the gorse was a brilliant yellow. The combination was breathtaking in the dry sunny weather, but I kept quiet as we drove home, letting Aidan and Carl exchange news of family and friends.

The visit went well enough, considering that it was January. Carlota complained of the mud on the roads and footpaths, which she called 'caca', never having encountered rural mud before. One rainy afternoon Carl decided to make rock cakes, causing total chaos in the kitchen and resulting in inedible, aptly named buns. He roared with laughter, delighted at the mess, and we fed the inedible cakes to the seagulls. Another day, when Aidan and I had left them asleep in the house, we came back to find a note on the kitchen table in Carl's child-like handwriting, 'Gone for a lovely walk!' It became a family joke, an oft-used formula, and a reminder of Carl's innate optimism. I was glad that he accepted me without question, not of course as a stepmother, he was already twenty-seven, but as a friend of his, as well as his father's new partner.

*

Soon after Carl and Carlota's visit, I heard on the grapevine that Frank Buckley was out for my blood. He was accusing me of taking his music manuscripts to the dump. I noticed that they had gone from the front hall, but it was nothing to do with me. I asked Aidan about the missing manuscript mountain, and he explained that he had got tired of looking at the untidy heap every time he came in and out, and had put them out for the bin men.

'But they were the Buck's compositions, didn't you think to ask him before you threw them out?' Apparently not – they had been there so long, Aidan had assumed they were discards.

Luckily Frank was able to trace them to the Civic Amenity Centre, as the dump was now called, and reclaim them before they were thrown into the incinerator. But he had assumed that I was the tidy one who threw things out, not Aidan. I asked Aidan to explain the facts to Frank and apologise, which he did. 'It wouldn't have happened to Beethoven!' was Frank's aggrieved complaint. He gave Aidan a bollocking, but somehow they ended up friends again.

Some weeks later, on St Valentine's night, Aidan and I were having dinner in Max's Wine Bar, our favourite restaurant in those days. No sooner had we taken our seats when someone lunged dramatically across the floor and threw himself on his knees in front of me. It was the Buck, pleading forgiveness for having made the terrible mistake of blaming me for the binning of his manuscripts. I assured him all was forgiven, and he kissed my hand in an operatic gesture.

Max's was a very small restaurant, and the other diners had watched this touching scene with interest, none more so than the couple at the next table. When Frank had finished, the man stood up and approached our table. I recognised the American author, Howard Simpson. He asked if he could introduce his wife, Mary Alice.

It was the start of a warm friendship between the four of us. The Simpsons were even older than Aidan, and had four daughters. Howard was a Californian of old stock, and Mary Alice had been born in Las Vegas before it had casinos. Howard was retired from the American Foreign Service. He was posted to Saigon in the early 1950s as adviser to the prime minister, and was present at the Battle of Dien Bien Phu. Other postings included Paris, Canberra and Algiers. But his favourite one was US Consul in Marseille, where one of his annual 'duties' was to attend the Cannes Film Festival – the opposite of a hardship posting, as he liked to observe. In his retirement he took up writing, alternating serious military history with potboilers featuring a French detective called Bastide, to supplement his pension. Locally he was said to be an undercover CIA agent.

Shortly after our meeting in Max's, a couple of Russian factory ships anchored up the river near the Simpsons' house, giving rise to a local rumour that they were there to keep an eye on the American 'spy' – that is to say, Howard.

Eventually I challenged Aidan on his public rubbishing of my work. He looked sheepish – a downward glance to the side, and an upward look through pleading eyes – and asked who had told me.

'Rourk.'

'Do you care that much what Rourk thinks of your work?'

'It's the principle. You shouldn't bad-mouth my work in front of other people.'

'That's a terrible expression, "bad-mouth". So is "rubbishing". You shouldn't use Americanisms.'

This was the start of a campaign to encourage me to talk – and therefore write – in a better way, less sloppy and slangy, more precise. Clichés, tired or not, were outlawed.

Words that I was told to eliminate from my vocabulary:

Loads of
Spectacular
Huge

Once he picked up on them, I was amazed at how often I used them in conversation. When I commented on this, 'amazed' was immediately added to the list.

To soften the criticism he told me a story about Jorge Luis Borges in Buenos Aires in 1927, shortly after a failed eye operation had left him totally blind. A friend offered to take him out for an evening with the young poets of Buenos Aires, how would he like that? Borges agreed to the excursion, and his friend took him to a quiet bar downtown. They had a few drinks and talked to various people. Then his friend suggested it was time to go home. 'But where are the young poets of Buenos Aires?' Borges asked.

'They were the people we've been talking to all evening.'

'Well, they didn't talk like poets,' said Borges.

One afternoon, when we were living in the house in Summercove, a Garda squad car parked on the quay, and Guard Paul Doyle knocked on our front door, looking for Aidan. I answered, and was intrigued. I left the pair of them in the kitchen, where they talked for about half an hour. Aidan then walked with him across the quay, and politely saw him into the squad car, closing the door for him.

'What was all that about?' I asked when he came back in.

'He wanted a formal statement about Colman's car crash.'

I looked blank. 'Car crash?'

'The last night I was there after Christmas, when you were in London. Colman drove out of the car park of Lil Doyle's pub at closing time without looking, and his car was hit by another one. It was a write-off. Luckily none of us were hurt, but Sylvia was a bit shaken up.'

'Why didn't you tell me about it?'

'I did, the first night you got back from London. We were in bed.'

'I was probably asleep.'

'Maybe so. I wondered why you didn't say anything.'

I introduced Aidan to my friends Katherine and Joachim Beug because I knew they would like one another. Katherine was an American artist, with Irish grandparents. She and Joachim, who was from Hamburg and twelve years older, had met at Northwestern University in Chicago. When he was offered a lectureship in the German department at University College Cork, Katherine urged him to accept. She had been to Kinsale when travelling as a student, and had been tempted to stay, so she decided they would live there, within commuting distance of the college.

Aidan had a liking for all things German, and he and Joachim became friends. At the Beug's house we met Joachim's friend, Gerry Wrixon, UCC's professor of micro-electronics, and his American wife, Marcia. Both Katherine and Marcia were strong women with opinions of their own, the sort of women Aidan liked, while Gerry and Joachim were also good, occasionally argumentative company.

For the first six months that he lived in Kinsale, Aidan got on well with everybody, including the poet

Desmond O'Grady. It was generally agreed that O'Grady was a handful, OK on a good day, but inclined to drink too much, and become overbearing. He cultivated the persona of a poet, always wore a dark red Kinsale smock (a long-sleeved canvas top with patch pockets across the lower front) and a black-and-white keffiyeh around his shoulders. His black hair was greying, and his face could politely be described as 'lived-in', being both wrinkled and scarred, but there were still the remnants of a good-looking charmer. Born near Limerick, he had gone to Paris after boarding school, and spent most of the 1950s in that city, living and working at the bookshop Shakespeare & Co., eventually meeting Picasso, Samuel Beckett, Sartre and de Beauvoir and whoever else you care to mention. His stories seemed outlandish, but were usually true, for example his claim to have lived in Venice as secretary and factotum to Ezra Pound and Olga Rudge. When his first collection of poetry was published in 1956, he had sent a copy to Ezra Pound in St Elizabeth's Psychiatric Hospital in Washington, D.C. Pound took one of the poems for his review, and on his return to Europe, O'Grady became his secretary. He spent most of the 1960s between Rome and Venice; Fellini gave him a cameo in *La Dolce Vita*, playing, inevitably, an Irish poet. His charmed existence included some years at Harvard as a teaching fellow, where he completed a PhD, a rare achievement for someone who had never been an undergraduate. He taught at American universities in Cairo and Alexandria, and spent summers in Greece, usually on the island of Paros. He moved back to Ireland, like Derek and Aidan, in the early 1980s when the establishment of Aosdána guaranteed him an income. He was a showman, had known many literary and artistic characters, and could be very entertaining; but he could also be a real pain in the arse when drunk. I preferred his girlfriend, Ellen Beardsley. She was in her late twenties, intense, seriously interested in Korean poetry, which she translated, as well as writing her own work. She was often very funny, and as mad about Desmond as I was about Aidan. They had met on Paros, and she was taking a break from a promising academic career to spend time in Ireland with Desmond – whom I always called Desmondo, as a nod to his well-travelled status.

We first met when Aidan ran into Ellen and Desmond one evening in January 1987 in our local pub, the Bulman. They were living in Desmond's cottage on a hill above the village, and had just got back from a long stay abroad. Aidan knew Desmond slightly, having given a reading with him and John Banville at the Poetry Society in London during the 'Sense of Ireland' cultural festival in 1980. Desmond's daughter had filmed the event, and from what I could gather from Aidan's account it seemed that Desmond had hogged the limelight, lying as if in his coffin, lit by tall candles, and taking more than his share of their allotted time. However, it seemed Aidan bore no grudge. We invited them to supper the night after we met, and they invited us the following week. Ellen disappeared after serving the meal, leaving Desmond to hold the floor and entertain us with anecdotes now over-familiar to her. Desmond showed us around his library. It seems he had known everybody – each book he pulled down contained a handwritten letter from the author, an exotic postcard or a newspaper clipping of a review. Among the names were Robert Lowell, Pablo Neruda, Yevgeny Yevtushenko, Allen Ginsberg, Dylan Thomas. It was the first time I had seen a library like this, and I was fascinated. Aidan was quietly sipping red wine,

O'Grady's tipple at this time of day. He kept large bottles of Valpolicella in his hot press beside the immersion heater. His cottage, while picturesque, could be cold and damp, even in summer.

Derek was surprised to hear about our convivial evening at Rincurran Cottage. He had not expected Aidan and Desmond to get on. Derek had known Desmond for much longer than Aidan. When Aidan dismissed Desmond's work as 'not interesting', Derek stood up for it, claiming that whatever about his personal manner, Desmond had published half a dozen very good poems, and you could not ask more than that of any poet. When Aidan actually got around to reading Desmond's work, he had to agree. He particularly like the poem 'Tipperary', with its reference to 'those Limerick Junctions of daily resolution'. Limerick Junction is a stop on the Cork–Dublin railway, way out in the middle of nowhere, where you change for the branch line to Limerick City. It was known for extremely long, unexplained delays.

★

Aidan and my father Denis, known as Pa in the family, got on well right from the start. Aidan refers to him in his diary early on as 'a jolly decent old cove'. I had told my father that Aidan had been a scratch golfer when he was younger, so my father immediately invited him for a round at Kinsale's nine-hole golf links. Pa admired his long, straight drives, and the accuracy of his putting. He had read *Images of Africa*, and commented on the similarities between the precision of Aidan's writing, his choice of exactly the right word, and the precision of his putting. Not inclined to chat himself, he enjoyed Aidan's quiet company. This was new territory for me – a boyfriend who could be friends with my father. Born in 1911, my father was only sixteen years older than Aidan. He had wanted to do an English degree before studying medicine, but he was one of six children, all needing professions, and the idea seemed an outlandish indulgence to his father, whom he quoted: 'If you're doing medicine, go and do medicine, none of this messing around with English. Plenty of time to read books once you're qualified.' Of course that was a lie, but Denis never lost his love of reading, especially George Eliot who was born in Nuneaton, near his home, nature writers and diarists like Richard Jefferies and Parson Woodforde, and English poetry. Like many people of his generation, A. P. Wavell's *Other Men's Flowers* was a favourite anthology. Every Christmas from the age of twelve I found a hefty poetry anthology, usually an Oxford one, among my presents, which soon found its way back into my father's hands. His career as a consultant anaesthetist, who also taught, with a wife and young daughter to entertain, did not leave much time for reading.

My mother, Angela, was not so easy to win over. Even before meeting Aidan, she had decided that he was too old for me, and was unreliable, having left a wife and three children. He obviously had no money. He could not even drive a car. But after meeting him, she seemed to soften. The Simpsons gave a drinks party for my parents, whom they knew slightly, inviting half a dozen other friends, most of them 'old colonial hands', who had retired to Kinsale after a career overseas. My mother felt at home in this elegant gathering of people, all of whom had a high opinion of Aidan.

After the party, we went for dinner to Jim Edwards' restaurant. Relaxing as we took our seats, Aidan started to tell them the story of how his youngest son Elwin was conceived in Dublin, because Jill's friend had forgotten to post the contraceptives from London. If I could have kicked him under the table I would have, but I was too far away. He went on, 'We even thought of an abortion, another child seemed an impossible prospect, but I'm so glad we went ahead, an abortion would have been a terrible mistake. Elwin is the most cheerful of all my sons, and he will go far.'

I had explained that my parents were practising Catholics, my father a convert from low Church of England, my mother the president of the Chelsea branch of the St Vincent de Paul Society: what was he thinking? Perhaps I was the only person listening to him: nobody else made any comment. My mother, whose mind was already fading, often lost track of Aidan's elaborate sentences, and quicksilver changes of topic, and would turn to my father and ask quietly: 'What's he on about now, dear?'

This became an expression I sometimes mimicked to tease Aidan when he got carried away by magnificent flights of fancy. 'What's he on about now, dear?'

My parents had made friends in Summercove, a Protestant couple of roughly their age. Ashley Good, from a well-known local farming family, had been a dashing young RAF pilot when he had married an Englishwoman, Joanna. They had stayed on in Egypt after the end of the war, where he worked as a flying instructor. In retirement he ran a ship chandlery in Kinsale, and pottered about in boats. Joanna never really settled in Ireland, and was known for having a sharp tongue and speaking her mind. She would have been much happier living on the south coast of England, and often said so. She and my mother, originally a native of Summercove, got on famously. When Joanna's face was disfigured by surgery for skin cancer, my mother arranged for her to come and stay with her in London and have special classes in make-up for cancer patients. The four of them had drinks together at least once a week, either at the Bulman, or at a smarter cocktail bar up the road in Scilly. Occasionally they went out to dinner together; neither Joanna nor Angela ever went to coffee mornings, a popular pastime with Kinsale ladies, nor did they meet on their own to go walking or shopping in Cork, only as a foursome.

My father found Aidan's insistence on the ingredients of his gin and tonic most amusing, and added to it, we never knew why, the stipulation that the glass should be cooled in the fridge beforehand. If we were coming over for a drink he would always say, 'Jolly good, I'll put a glass in the fridge for Aidan.'

The Higgins Gin and Tonic is actually quite simple: Gordon's gin, Schweppes tonic, slice of lemon, some ice. But in Cork people prefer Cork Dry Gin, Schweppes is not universally available in pubs, ditto lemon, and out in the country ice used to be a rarity. If you ask for Gordon's, a bottle can usually be found, but the same is not true of Schweppes tonic. On one occasion, lemon cordial was offered instead of a lemon slice. Ice used to be a problem, but nowadays it can usually be found, if you insist. I remember in particular a small country pub on a very hot afternoon. The elderly woman tending the bar walked, with difficulty, a considerable distance into the back quarters of the pub, and returned with a slice of lemon on a saucer. 'And ice? Is there any ice?' She looked at him despairingly, and when he did not relent, she stoically repeated the trek, to return some minutes later with two ice cubes melting on the saucer.

★

The Great Patrician Scholar had set herself a deadline of 17 March to finish the first draft of the St Patrick book, and she made it, just. These were pre-computer days: as I finished each chapter I passed it on to Ellen, who could type, and was glad of the money. She retyped it, ready for copying. She delivered the 280 pages to me as a gift-wrapped package, a huge brick of white paper decorated with green ribbons and orange crocuses.

St Patrick's Day was a holiday, but I avoided all celebrations. Aidan and I walked around Compass Hill, one of our favourite town walks, calling in for a drink with Derek en route. It was a long time since we'd had a walk together, as I'd been concentrating on the book. It was a mild day, clear and sunny, and for the first time, I noticed that the daffodils and primroses were out. It was wonderful to contemplate a St Patrick-free evening which could be spent playing Scrabble and reading a novel. I felt fresher than I had for a long time, but a bit dazed, as if I had burnt up a large quantity of brain cells.

I knew it was a first draft, and would need more work, but I was pleased to have it done after a solid six months' writing since October. I had even weathered the drastic change from single person to couple, with only minor interruptions to my writing schedule. But Aidan saw that I was unhappy when I should have been elated at finishing the huge chore. I explained that I had run out of money.

'How much do you need?'

'£1,500 would do.'

'I'll raid my deep savings. I have about £4,000 stashed away. What's mine is yours.'

'Not to worry, I'll manage. I've started reviewing again. And the payment on delivery will be in any day.'

Of course it wasn't. But I managed. And I really appreciated his offer. His deep savings must have survived many a crisis in the three years since he'd earned the money teaching in Texas, and I admired him for keeping them intact. He had not even thought of raiding them to pay off his double overdraft. He had a buoyantly optimistic view of his finances: his diaries are full of lists of money owed to him for various ventures, most of which came to nothing: pieces submitted to the *London Magazine*, which he assumed would be accepted, reviews commissioned at his request by *The Spectator*, the *Irish Times*, *The Guardian*, the *Financial Times* which were returned as 'unusable', due to his idiosyncratic, elliptical style. The radio play *Assassin* had been submittted to BBC Northern Ireland, and he was still waiting for the Abbey's verdict on the stage play of the same name.

Aidan's attitude to freelance work as an established writer of high literary repute was very different from my approach. I was a member of the National Union of Journalists, an active trade unionist, a firm believer in the power of collective bargaining and in maintaining professional standards. When I started reviewing again after finishing the first draft of the St Patrick book, I was complaining one day about having to rush a review of a Rebecca West novel into the post without being totally happy with it. Aidan commented that he never sent off a review unless he was completely sure of it. He'd rather miss a deadline than send out something substandard. That made me feel like a terrible hack. But then he was a writer, not a journalist. He had other sources of income – the radio plays earned as much as a novel back then – £4,000[*] was not unusual, and then there were repeat fees – and he was getting royalties from John Calder again, thanks

---

[*] Worth about £12,000 today.

to Reg. But he was much less realistic than I was when it came to calcuating future income, adding work he hadn't yet got around to writing, to the final figure. I admired his blithe optimism, but soon learnt that he was far worse with money than I was.

Still, we shared the belief that 'What's mine is yours'. While we retained separate bank accounts, we never had a single disagreement about money. If one of us (usually but not always Aidan) had more cash to hand than the other, then the one who had the money paid more, and so it came and went.

★

I took Aidan on a tour of west Cork while we waited for Grafton to respond. We had a couple of days of glorious idleness in Allihies, a former mining village on the rocky edge of west Cork, talking to the old folk in the three pubs. It reminded Aidan of Inishere back in 1952. There was also a kitchen-table round of catching up with various friends: the philosopher Norman Steele and his wife, Veronica, of Milleens farmhouse cheese fame, the sculptor and geologist Cormac Boydell and his artist wife Rachel Parry, and the artist and musician Tim Goulding, whose father had bought a treasured Patrick Collins painting from Aidan some twenty years earlier, when he was in dire need of money. I had used one of Tim's Allihies landscapes for the cover of *The Out-haul* back in 1985. His wife Annie's copy of *Bornholm Night-Ferry* was presented for signature (she was away working as ship's cook on the sail-training ship, the *Asgard*). Aidan had been to Tim's recent show at the Taylor Galleries in Dublin: everyone knew everyone else, and we all liked each other's work and way of living, and the sun never stopped shining. Or so it seemed.

Grafton took a long time to react, and meanwhile there was no cheque in the post. Once I had done my allotted reviewing, I spent my time either writing a long-form piece for Aidan about living in Mexico in the 1970s which might also evolve into a short story, or reading Beckett and Higgins. The dry humour and playfulness of *Murphy* was a delightful revelation to me, its erudition an enjoyable challenge. Eventually I heard from Reg. Grafton wanted revisions to 'popularise' the book, and asked for more emphasis on Americans and St Patrick's Day. They disliked my title, *St Patrick and the Irish People*, and intended to replace it with *The Living Legend of St Patrick*. The word 'legend' made me cringe: I myself would never buy a book with 'Legend' in the title. Worse still, until these revisions were done and approved, there would be no payment on delivery. Instead of the long-awaited large cheque which I had worked so hard for, I was told that a detailed letter from my Grafton editor would follow.

Aidan was furious on my behalf. His advice was to dig in my heels, stick out for my title, and refuse to do anything more than minor revisions. Better still, why did I not just abandon it, give it up as a bad job, and go back to writing stories?

'But then I would lose a whole year's work, and I'd have to pay back the advance. That would be a disaster, a total waste.'

'Nothing is ever wasted,' he said, an oft-repeated mantra. 'You can find another publisher for the book, a more serious one.'

Effectively, he was advising me to begin again. I could not face that prospect, and neither could I pay back the money I had already been paid. Better to deal with what I had in hand, get the book out, and the money in the bank.

The Grafton letter didn't arrive for about ten days, and meanwhile there was another long phone call from Reg in which he used all his considerable charm to persaude me to do what had been asked of me. Eventually I conceded that he and Grafton knew more than I did about what sold, therefore I would agree to the new title, and all the revisions. 'Don't forget all those Irish-Americans,' he said. 'We're not talking real money at all yet...'

Meanwhile I had reread the typescript, and started to see a way to make the book lighter and more attractive to casual readers. The letter from Grafton was not much help; my plan, which involved putting more emphasis on the travel writing and less on the history, was better. I buckled down and did a substantial rewrite (but no new research), completing it in two weeks. This time the coffers were so empty that I had to do my own typing, which invloved much cutting and pasting (literally – using scissors and glue – the lines between stuck-on text and the new page disappeared when photocopied), but I didn't mind. Anything to get it off my desk, the cheque in the bank, and regain the freedom to write whatever I liked.

*

I was so immersed in the St Patrick book and the arrival of Aidan that I hadn't noticed there had been a long silence from the Arts Council about my application to join Aosdána. Then one morning in late April Aidan mentioned that his mail contained an appalling letter from the poet John Jordan, among the nominations for membership, urging him to vote for someone whom Jordan was proposing. So where was my application for membership? We checked the papers that had been circulated to members, and there was nothing there from Ernie or Derek. Neither Ernie, Derek nor I had heard anything since sending off the package the previous September, but none of us had thought to query the silence.

Derek got on the phone. Adrian Munnelly, the Registrar of Aosdána, was most apologetic that no one had got back to him or to Ernie; there had been an oversight. But the *Toscaireacht*, the committee of members who vetted applications before circulating the names of proposed new members, had decided not to put my name forward. They did not need to give any reason, but perhaps, the registrar suggested, I was not well known enough in Ireland, or perhaps my work was not considered a substantial enough 'corpus'. Yet people less well known than me had readily been admitted, and people with a smaller body of published work too. But usually they were Dublin-based. It was all too easy to speculate that my application had been turned down at the first hurdle because I lived in Kinsale, was published in London, had an English education, and did not 'work the room' in Dublin. Or perhaps it was because Ernie was disliked in the wake of his divorce from Edna O'Brien?

At one blow, and with not even an official letter to show for it, my dream of having a regular income that would allow me to work on my fiction full-time was shattered. I wrote to Ernie to let him know, as no one from the Arts Council had done so. We were all puzzled at this rejection, but none of us wanted to pursue it any further, especially me. Perhaps if I had also submitted my poetry to small reviews published in Ireland, my name would have gone further. I did my best to put this bizarre rejection out of my mind, and get on with life. And writing.

But it is not easy, being rejected. I woke up early on Sunday morning furious, and found myself dissolving in tears of rage. Aidan hugged me gently and asked what was wrong. When I explained he said, 'Is that all that's the matter? I thought you were crying about something important, that you'd decided you and I didn't really like each other, that you were just pretending.' I got over it. The way forward lay in working harder, writing better and publishing more. While I was waiting for the next tranche of my St Patrick money, I was already working full-time on my piece about Mexico City that I had promised Aidan. It was going well, and Aidan and I were happy with each other. That was all that mattered.

★

I had known Peter Murray, the Director of the Crawford Municipal Art Gallery in Cork, ever since moving to Kinsale in 1982. Coincidentally, Peter's sister, Catherine Murray, was writing her MA dissertation at the Sorbonne on *Langrishe, Go Down*, so naturally I introduced him to Aidan. Peter and his wife, Sarah Iremonger, an artist in her early twenties, often spent time in Kinsale at weekends, with us or with Derek or Stan. After a particularly heated argument with Aidan about the artist Seán Keating (a twentieth-century realist whose work he loathed), Peter turned to me and said, 'Aidan does not approach an argument with an open mind. He is like a soldier going over the ridge into battle with a fixed bayonet.' I liked that; the image stayed with me for a long time.

★

One evening, while I was cooking at the Summercove house, the phone rang in the hall adjoining the kitchen, and I answered it. A woman with a strange English accent asked for Aidan in a very proprietorial tone. I suspected it was Jill.

She sounded nice. I closed the kitchen door and let Aidan take his phone call in private.

When we went over to the pub for a nightcap, Aidan told me the woman on the phone was Mary, the protagonist of his story 'The Bird I Fancied'. Of course, it was not a South African accent, it was a west of England one, with cockney overtones from years of living in London. He was impressed, because after two years of believing himself in love with her, he felt nothing when he heard her voice on the phone. He said he had been thinking of her the day we walked in Garrettstown Woods, looking for bluebells, because he had once had her in a bluebell wood. That stung, he hadn't needed to tell me that, but I didn't say so. Instead, I said perhaps it was time we started to acknowledge the existence of *amor* between us. He agreed, saying he thought it was definitely there, that was obvious, but he was superstitious about naming it, declaring it, in case it went away. To which I replied, 'My sentiments exactly.' And there we left the subject. I understood his reluctance to introduce a ritual of declarations of love, and approved of his decision. He acted as if he loved me, and that was what mattered – show, don't tell. I also knew that you do not form a relationship with a brilliant, unconventional man and then complain because he does not follow the conventional pattern. We loved each other, we both knew it, and there was no need to be constantly affirming it.

The Mary business made me realise how much I cared about Aidan, how possessive I had become in such a short time (four months), and also how complacent – assuming I was the only woman he ever thought about. And also of course I realised how much I could be hurt – inevitable, if one is going to fall in love.

★

The Aosdána disaster was followed by the news that Aidan's publisher, Allison and Busby, was in liquidation. So instead of having two books out this year, he would have none. Then came word from BBC Northern Ireland that they were not going to take his radio play *Assassin*, as it too closely resembled *Franz Ferdinand*, a play by Aidan already produced by BBC London. *The Spectator* had returned his review apologetically, with a one-line note on a compliments slip saying it was 'unusable'. Aidan's gnomic, often elliptical style did not lend itself to mainstream reviewing. And a review he had sent to the *Irish Times* was apparently lost in the post. The next morning Aidan woke up and said, 'Nobody is publishing what I write, the BBC won't broadcast my plays, the *Irish Times* has lost my reviews. I might as well stay in bed with Zinnia.'

Talking in Bed

We were talking about depressing place names, arguing about whether Morden, at the southern end of the Northern Line, was worse than Lurgan, a town in County Armagh. Dalston, Frognal, Elmer's End. Ballyhaunis, Birr, Bunratty, Kinnegad, Athy, Moyle, Mogeely. And there were beautiful place names, Newbliss in Monaghan, rechristened *Nouvelle Exstase* by some poet, and Morelia in central Mexico, then Chimborazo, Cotopaxi, Zihuatanejo, Mixcoac, Sayulita...

That night we couldn't sleep, so we started making up a story lying in the dark, contributing alternate lines: 'There were two dog-rough bachelor farmers, Morden and Lurgan, who shared the family home.'

'Their life was complicated because they were both in love with the same woman, a beauty by the name of Morelia...'

'She lived in the nearest village, Ballyhaunis…'

We must have talked ourselves to sleep, because I can't remember any more.

One Saturday morning, when we were still staying in the house by the sea, Aidan went down to the kitchen around midday and saw his brother's face through the window, leaning a piece of paper on it while he wrote a note. On opening the door, Aidan saw the new Mini that Colman had bought to replace the one that had been wrecked in the late-night crash last December, and Sylvia huddled in the backseat. Because he often used the car as a van, to transport buiding materials for the ongoing work on his house, Colman had removed the front seat of the Mini, relegating Sylvia to the back one. It was Colman's birthday, and he and Sylvia had decided to drive the four hours from Wicklow to Kinsale to see Aidan's new base. They had not let us know of their intention, not wanting to cause any bother. I was summoned from upstairs, and introduced to a most unusual couple. Colman was very thin, a much wirier build than Aidan, and taller. He wore ancient corduroy trousers, a tight-fitting Fair Isle sweater under a worn and patched tweed jacket, its top pocket lined with sharp pencils. He was clean-shaven under uncombed grey hair, and had the sweetest smile I had ever seen – very like Aidan's. Though he was two years younger than Aidan, he looked years older. He was thinner and fairer with a higher voice. There was something ethereal about him.

Sylvia, a slight woman of medium height, with wispy grey hair that still had streaks of blonde, had a lovely smile too. She was possibly the strangest woman I'd ever met. She wore a long tweed skirt under an ancient three-quarter-length cardigan in a shade of beige that she referred to as 'oatmeal'. The cardigan was patched and darned all over, as was what could be seen of the skirt. They could have walked out of an illustration for a Depression-era novel.

Aidan immediately invited them in, and I made coffee. Colman wanted to find out first-hand details of the statement that Aidan had made to the gardaí about the car accident, as it could affect his insurance claim. They had been phoning us since 11 a.m., but they were ringing the phone at the Dutch House. Eventually Stan had answered, and told them where to find us. I would have liked to make them lunch, but we had no food in the house, having not yet gone into Kinsale for the weekly shop, so Aidan ushered us into the Bulman for a drink. The three of them had gin and tonic, as a birthday celebration. It is not a drink I have ever liked: I stuck to Coke. It was noisy in the Bulman, being Saturday lunchtime, but not yet warm enough to take our drinks outside onto the quay. Colman, an architect, wanted to see the new village of holiday homes at Castlepark, which had recently won a major award. I told him it was just across the harbour. 'I can't see any village,' he said, and I explained that its invisibility from most vantage points on the outer harbour was one reason why it had won the award. I offered to drive them across, to give them a rest from the car after their long journey. We were also hoping that the Dock Bar on the other side of the harbour would be quieter, and might manage some food.

We walked all around the small cluster of houses, from the Dock Bar in front to the sandy beach behind it, Colman admiring the ingenuity of the architects, with the differing roof pitches and the use of traditional slates and whitewash. The pub was blissfully quiet, and Nora, the obliging *bean an tí* (or landlady), made a big plate of cheese-and-tomato sandwiches. Colman and Sylvia had been vegetarians for many years, and according to Aidan lived off cheese omelettes and apple pie. I suggested to Sylvia that she take a seat on a bar stool. 'No thank you. I'm practising standing.' I think it was meant to be a joke. Sylvia was so respectful of all living things that she had recently persuaded Colman to get rid of the water-butt from which he watered the garden because it was a death-trap for slugs. After taking a good close look at me, she told Aidan that I reminded her of brother B, as he and Colman called their elder brother, Brendan. This was puzzling to Colman and Aidan: the only thing Brendan and I had in common was black hair. That was presumably enough for Sylvia. I drove us all back around the harbour to Summercove, and offered them a bed for the night, and dinner. But as suddenly as they had arrived, Colman and Sylvia got back into their three-seated Mini and headed up the hill at the start of their four-hour return journey to Wicklow. I liked Colman very much, especially when he relaxed and started talking. I found it easy to make him laugh; we seemed to get on well. He and Aidan were obviously very fond of each other, more like twins than just brothers.

*

A few weeks after Colman's visit, Reg phoned to say that Grafton had accepted my revised manuscript, and my cheque would be in the post. At last I was through with St Patrick: all I had to do was correct the proofs and plan the launch. I took Aidan out to dinner at his friend Jim Edwards' bar and we celebrated with sole on the bone (me) and roast duck (him).

Aidan's friend Fiona Adamczewski wrote to say that she was flying into Cork Airport to visit some friends in Kerry. Could he book her a B&B in Kinsale for a night, before she went on to Kerry? We booked her into Jimmie's. We had met and liked our neighbour Jimmie Conron, who lived in the old Parochial House with his widowed father, and ran it as a B&B in the tourist season. He also played mandolin and sang with a guitar-playing friend in several bars around town. He was roughly the same age as Aidan's son Carl, and they had got on very well on his visit. Jimmie's B&B, which was across the road from the Dutch House and below Desmond Castle, became our B&B of choice for visiting friends.

I had met Fiona briefly earlier in the year when we went to London for a meeting with Robin Robertson, who was to become Aidan's editor at Secker & Warburg. We had also gone to the launch of Jill's novel, *McDaid's Wife*, a lightly fictionalised account of the time when she walked out on Aidan in Berlin during his affair with Hannelore, leaving him to take care of the three small boys. The launch was at a pub in Putney. When we walked into the room, Aidan was embraced warmly by a slim, very attractive woman with a loud South African voice: 'There you are, you old devil! Let's have a look at the new girlfriend!' Her remark, far from embarrassing me, was the perfect way to break the ice, and meant I didn't have to be formally introduced to Jill or anyone else. Everyone had a good look, I did my best to smile warmly, as if accepting a round of applause, and after the initial sudden silence, everyone started talking again.

Fiona was Jill's best friend from school, and they had taken the boat together aged twenty-two from South Africa to London in 1952. By then, Fiona (née Doran, her father was from Sligo) had a degree in history of art, while Jill, whose father could not afford to send her to university, had qualified as a secretary. Fiona's husband, Bernhard Adamczewski, had been a close friend of Aidan's when he was living in South Africa and London, and encouraged his writing. Adam, as he was known, was the model for the crafty eternal student, Otto Beck, in *Langrishe, Go Down*. In addition to her knowledge of art, Fiona was an avid reader of Beckett and the *TLS*, a founder member of the Hazlitt Society, a brilliant cook and party-giver, and enviably stylish. She and Adam had hosted the memorable party held shortly after the publication of *Langrishe, Go Down* in London in 1966, attended by Samuel Beckett.

The one day we had with Fiona in Kinsale turned out to be sunny, so we took her on a drive to the Old Head and beyond. She and I got on well. We walked around the ruined Franciscan abbey on the water's edge in Timoleague, talking all the while. I could sense that Aidan, who was not interested in ruins, was feeling sidelined: I had taken over his friend, and she was more interested in me than in him. It was time we went for a drink somewhere, and paid him some attention. I linked his arm, and as there were three pubs in the village, I asked:

'Where would you like your gin and tonic?'

'In my mouth.'

I dropped his arm, took one step away, gave him a cold look, then asked in a calm but unfriendly tone:

'Would you like to walk home?'

Fiona told me that was the moment when she knew I was the right woman for Aidan, and would be able to handle his difficult behaviour. 'Unlike Jill,' she said, 'who would have made a big scene, with tears and insults.'

Aidan had these occasional moments, usually with those closest to him, when he could be downright unpleasant. What to call it? Snarky? Nastier than that. He would often regret it after, and apologise. It was so unlike his usual gentle, courteous manner. The best way to describe it seemed the old Irish saw, that a devil got into him. His friend Dermot Healy had a devil in him too from time to time. Even I have a devil on occasion – maybe we all do?

★

Now that I was free to read again, I started catching up on the books that Aidan had brought with him from Wicklow. I picked up David Thomson's *Woodbrook* and hardly moved from my armchair until it was finished. Aidan took the battered paperback out of my hands.

'I see you read a book straight through, from beginning to end.'

'Well, yes. Doesn't everyone?'

'No. Only dull people read a book straight through. What you do is you look at the opening shot – "I was eighteen when I first saw Woodbrook." Excellent. Hard to beat a simple declarative sentence. Then you go to the ending: "There were only a few words in the letter. It said what I knew it would say when I picked it up from the mat – that Phoebe was dead." Excellent again!'

'But that way you know the ending!'

'Do you really keep reading just to find out what happened next?'

He had me there. Whatever answer I gave would be wrong. It was like 'When did you stop beating your wife?' I was starting to learn that living with Aidan was a constant challenge, a challenge to my fixed ideas and to received wisdom, to the habits of a lifetime. He had a most unusual mind and for all the jokes, he was never anything less than serious.

★

In early June we had moved back to our apartment in the Dutch House, as my parents were spending summer in the house in Summercove.

One morning in mid-June, shortly before Bloomsday, the public phone in the hallway of the Dutch House rang. It was *You* magazine of the *Mail on Sunday* looking for Stan. I also wrote for *You* magazine occasionally. 'He's away,' I said, 'Why don't you try me?' It worked: I was commissioned to go to Dublin, all expenses paid, to interview a film animator at 4 p.m. on Tuesday, write the copy up overnight, and telex it to London on Wednesday morning. Suddenly I was catapulted from my quiet life in a backwater into the heart of the metropolis. Who did I know in Dublin with a telex? I assembled the necessary amount of coins and rang Tim Magennis, Bord Fáilte's PR man, who had become a good friend after many a merry press trip, and he agreed to let me use his telex. There was an anxious wait for the interview to be confirmed, which happened just in time for us to drive to Cork and catch the evening train to Dublin. Aidan had decided to come with me.

I had booked a room at the Clarence, which, before it was bought by U2 and given a boomtime makeover, was a slightly shabby and pleasantly old-fashioned hotel much favoured by culchies, being roughly midway between Heuston Station, where trains from Cork and Galway arrived, and the city centre. I loved its art deco façade on the Liffey, and had been determined to stay there at some point. Now, thanks to the *Mail on Sunday*, I could.

Up to then I had never been in the front door of the Clarence, only the back one on a dingy cobbled street in Temple Bar, which led to its panelled back bar, where the *Irish Times*' literary editor, Brian Fallon, hosted a monthly sandwich lunch for his contributors. It was mainly attended by older men, a group that one of my writer friends referred to as 'the crypto-fascists'. Among the changing faces, Benedict Kiely, James Plunkett, Tony Cronin and Tony O'Riordan (a local history buff) were regulars. I wasn't sure if the label referred to their politics or was an in-joke that I didn't get. To me they were simply a group of interesting characters who enjoyed talking about books and sharing literary gossip.

Aidan booked dinner at Blazes, a bistro a short walk from the hotel, where he had had some good times in the past. On this night it was cold, almost empty, a dark, oddly decorated room, a relic of the 1970s. The so-called background music was loud and atrocious. Aidan asked for it to be turned down, but gradually the volume crept back up. We had avocado-and-walnut salad, chicken Kiev, then profiteroles. Back at the Clarence we had one nightcap in the bar, carefully avoiding a thin, crafty-looking man who kept eyeing us across the room, and seemed anxious to talk.

Next morning an apologetic phone call from the *Mail on Sunday* informed me that the interview had been cancelled. I was told to go over to the animation company's office and see if the animator could be persuaded to change his mind. He could not, greatly to my relief. I had little idea of who I was supposed to be interviewing or why. After ten years as a freelance journalist, I had developed the habit of leaving such details to the last minute. The magazine's commissioning editor apologised profusely for sending me up to Dublin for nothing and offered me a reasonable £200 kill fee, plus expenses. With all the excitement I had forgotten that I would be entitled to that.

It was 16 June, Bloomsday, and the 'crypto-fascists' were meeting in the back bar of the Clarence. No one was planning to attend any of the Bloomsday events, which were dismissed as 'all rubbish'. The choice was a discussion between Anthony Cronin and Francis Stuart in the early evening, or a dramatised reading of Molly Bloom's soliloquy later on. The idea, dreamt up between the Tourist Board and the Arts Council, of making a big fuss about Bloomsday on 16 June, the day described in *Ulysses* – which they pronounced Ulyss-*sayz* rather than Ulyss-*eez*, as I had always done – was never going to catch on, they said. The projected annual celebration of Joyce's novel was dismissed as doomed to failure. For a start, hardly anyone read it these days: it was 'terribly over-rated'. The conversation turned to more interesting topics.

I wanted to take advantage of this unexpected trip to Dublin and its accompanying windfall to buy some clothes, so we headed off on foot to Grafton Street. We returned to the Clarence via the Long Hall, which Aidan introduced as one of his father's favourite Dublin pubs. I found it gloomy and unenticing, a sad daytime drinking den. But I was enjoying being shown around by Aidan, who knew Dublin so much better than I did. Up to now we had mostly been on my territory.

We had an early supper at Nico's, a rather ordinary Italian restaurant in Dame Street. Ulick O'Connor was eating there alone, and Aidan, who knew him but didn't like him, carefully chose a table that was out of his sightline. This was just as well, because on a previous visit to Dublin, to attend a book launch in the Shelbourne Hotel hosted by my then publisher, Hamish Hamilton, Ulick had threatened the English writer Robert Nye (a fellow Hamish Hamilton author I had run into on the Dublin train) with fisticuffs for taking advantage of Charlie Haughey's tax exemption scheme. He very nearly knocked Robert down the stairs. Alarmed at this unprovoked aggression from an apparent madman, being unaware of Ulick's reputation as a sportsman and respected author, Robert and I had jumped straight into a taxi and returned to Heuston Station for the last train back to Cork.

After the meal Aidan and I walked up to Stephen's Green, and he showed me the Garden for the Blind, which he had been telling me about the previous week. I thought it was a wonderful idea, a garden that you could smell and touch, with plant labels in Braille. The reality was much smaller than I expected, a square enclosure, with just one wooden bench, heavily scented by lavender, the only flower in bloom. But it was nice that he had remembered to show it to me.

As we left the Green, Aidan pointed out the place where he had once seen Siobhán McKenna feeding the ducks. He was in awe of her beauty on stage, but said that in person her features were too big for conventional beauty; they were best seen from the middle of the stalls. Whenever he mentioned her, he recalled her having to be restrained from throwing herself into Micheál Mac Liammóir's grave, which seemed to Aidan the height of romance. She had died aged sixty-three the previous November, a few days before Aidan and I met. There was a kind of magic in walking across the Green in the long summer evening with someone who had so many memories of Dublin, gazing at the bright lights of the stately Shelbourne Hotel.

We didn't cross over to the hotel, but continued on the same side of the street to a bar called the Pembroke Lounge. Soon after we had settled with our drinks, I noticed a small, untidy man come in the emergency exit, and stand there, swaying to and fro, staring around the room. He was greeted warmly by Aidan as Michael Hartnett. As soon as the poet started talking, his appearance and insobriety were forgotten, and I was riveted. He told us he was translating the poems of the Spanish mystic St John of the Cross into both Irish and English, at the same time, if I understood correctly. He had a new collection coming out in July, *A Necklace of Wrens* – we must come to the launch. He asked after Derek Mahon, and said he was the best around – best poet presumably. He left soon after, with a distracted air, saying that he hadn't meant to stop, he was looking for someone who owed him money. We moved on for one drink at the Horseshoe Bar in the Shelbourne, feeling the need of a little luxury on what had turned into a cold, rainy evening.

Aidan insisted on a taxi back to the Clarence, for my sake, he said. I enjoyed going in the front door as a resident, and we were heading for the lift when a merry hubbub from the bar sent us both in the other direction – just for the one nightcap. We were spotted by the man we had successfully avoided the night before, who had the look of a freeloader. He introduced himself as Wilf, and told us that he had been a bullfighter in Mysore, a friend of Hemingway and Ava Gardner when both were broke, and had regularly performed a perfect half-Veronica. He'd spent some time in Auschwitz as a child, and when chess was mentioned, he told us that he had once played Spassky and lost. He had money, contrary to our assumption, and bought us a drink. I noticed he had holes in his sweater, and asked if he had recently been gored by a bull. He saw the joke, and we parted friends. We retired at about one in the morning, after ordering papers and a pot of coffee to our room for 9 a.m. from the night porter. He had seen the man we had been talking to, and told us he's quite harmless, just an ex-jockey who'd landed on his head once too often.

The next day Aidan had arranged a visit to Springfield in Celbridge, his childhood home, and the house he had recreated in words as the setting for *Langrishe, Go Down*, and the inspiration for much of his writing. It seemed perfectly normal to Aidan that the current owners, a commercial pilot, Alistair Campbell and his wife, Rachel, who had put the property on the market (a 'small shooting box' as the auctioneer's advertisement quaintly called it), should invite him for a courtesy visit before they moved on. To me it was very exciting to be taking the Birr bus from Eden Quay, as Helen does in the long opening scene of *Langrishe*, to visit the fabled demesne: 'The lights in the bus burned dim, orange-hued behind opaque bevelled glass; ranged below the luggage racks they lit up the advertisement panels with repeated circles of bilious light.'

But we were travelling on a sunny summer day, and the 11.20 bus from Eden Quay was a well-ventilated double-decker. The destination those days was Edenderry, not the more distant Birr. We bagged the front seat on the upper deck, which only added to my excitement. I love bus journeys, especially new ones. By Conyngham Road it already felt as if we were out of the city, the leaves on the tall trees the freshest of greens, passing names familiar to me chiefly from Aidan's writing: Chapelizod, Lucan, then a narrow leafy lane where Aidan pointed out Donycomper, the graveyard visited by Helen in *Langrishe*. Then the bus crossed a twisted bridge and arrived in the village of Celbridge. Aidan showed me the National School that he had attended for only one day, and the place where he had waded across the river in a flood. We got off the bus in a sudden rush of excitement, Celbridge at last, and walked up towards the gates of Castletown House and into a pub called the Castletown Inn.

We were meeting Bernard Share there, the editor of the Aer Lingus magazine *Cara*, whom I knew already, having written a cover story about Cobh for his magazine the year before. Bernard, a man of letters, with a passion for words, and a musician, had published a couple of novels, and was an old friend of Aidan's. He had answered Aidan's letters packed with questions about Dublin topography when he was writing *Langrishe* in Johannesburg, and had given *Langrishe* a much-quoted laudatory review in the *Irish Times* when it first came out, writing that it was 'clearly the best novel by an Irish writer since *At Swim-Two-Birds* and the novels of Beckett'. No wonder Bernard had become a friend for life.

But I was puzzled as to how he fitted in to this excursion. Aidan had failed to explain that Bernard and his wife Elizabeth, along with Bernard's harmonium, lived in an apartment that had been created on the ground floor of Springfield. The Campbell's sale of the house meant that the Shares also had to find a new home, and they were in the midst of buying and renovating a house in a nearby village, Sallins. Bernard was surprised to hear that we were buying a house in Kinsale. 'Settling down?' he asked Aidan, in apparent disbelief. 'Yes. Enough of living in other people's houses.' Bernard was curious about Kinsale, and our being able to live there. He would have preferred a house on the sea, and could only tolerate Sallins because it was on a canal, from which he could travel all the way to the Shannon on his canal boat, and hence out into the wider world. It was also close to Elizabeth's job as a technical translator, and handy enough for the Aer Lingus offices at Dublin airport. Bernard had two sons in Australia, and the main reason he worked for Aer Lingus was the perk of subsidised travel: he loved to travel almost as much as he loved music and Elizabeth.

Springfield was even more beautiful than I had expected: 'idyllic' seemed the appropriate word on a perfect midsummer day. When we took our seats in Bernard's sitting room, Aidan immediately said, 'A winter evening, shelves of books there, the Da there, the Ma here,' pointing to either side of the fire, in such a matter-of-fact way, as if they were physically there. The large bay window looked out across a bed of flowering roses to a giant sycamore, already a big tree when Aidan was a child. He said the sycamore had a very special smell, close-to.

Bernard went to his study to work, and we took our glasses of wine out to the garden. Swallows were flying low past the window, 'A sign of rain,' said Aidan, leading me to the stables, where the swallows had their nests. The stables were unpainted, full of junk and lumber, the sky visible through the unglazed back window. He pointed to a recess where his father used to keep the Overlander, now covered with sensational dark pink and gold honeysuckle, climbing the height of the left-hand wall, alive with buzzing bees. Then we walked through a wooden door set in a stone wall and followed a path under a large, spreading yew tree, whose lower branches caught in my hair as I walked, and out on to a lawn the size of a tennis court – which it had once been – and beyond it a magnificent flower garden: tall pink lupins in clumps, randomly seeded foxgloves, and banks of smaller plants about to come into bloom, opposite a well-organised vegetable bed. We could hear but not see a gardener chipping away at something. To our right was a rustic bridge that crossed two small lily ponds and the path continued through a shrubbery. There was a timeless beauty to the garden that perfectly complemented the compact, unshowy Georgian house – or hunting box, as the current auctioneer's advertisement had it. The seventy-two acres that Aidan's father had sold with it in 1941 were now reduced to twelve.

Alistair and Rachel had spotted us in the stable yard and came out to introduce themselves. Alistair was a slim, grey-haired man in his mid-fifties with a boyish face. Rachel wore the countrywoman's uniform at the time: green wellies, a quilted waistcoat and a headscarf, rather like the Queen of England off-duty. They were both most welcoming to Aidan, showing us over the shrubbery, purple orchids scattered everywhere, tall dark-blue drumhead primulas rising above the ground cover. The background birdsong was intense, but the idyll was suddenly broken by a jumbo jet coming in to land. 'It doesn't often happen,' said Rachel, 'and after a while you don't notice.' She complained that the goldfish had been stolen by the Castletown herons. Aidan and Alistair talked about stone walls, and what was where in Aidan's day. We looked at the roller, still parked under the elm where Aidan had last seen it in 1941, its elaborate wrought-iron handle rusty but intact. Alistair and Rachel had restored the garden from a virtual wilderness in the seventeen years they had been in the house. They were moving back to England, to a smaller house in the West Country, a necessary economy with Alistair's retirement looming. But the house had failed to sell at auction earlier in the week. Rachel told Aidan that she cried that morning because they were selling Springfield, and she cried in the afternoon because it had not sold.

We went inside for a cup of tea. Two small dogs sat on the window seats in the front sitting room. It was decorated in quiet good taste, some modest antiques alongside newer pieces. Their daughter's batiks were hung in the carpeted corridors. A full set of servants' bells were still high up in the corridor outside the kitchen. Aidan was invited to show me around, and he took me up to the nursery, a twin-bedded room under the eaves overlooking the front paddock, that he had shared with Colman. The view of Dublin's mountains was now obscured by the growth of trees, which also hid the road past the front of the house and the electricity pylons. His mother's bedroom now had a bath installed in one corner, to avoid losing another room to a bathroom. Otherwise it was exactly as he remembered it.

When the Campbells heard that we intended to buy a house, and that I was keen on gardening, they offered us all sorts of cuttings, so that Aidan could take a bit of Springfield to his new home. Meanwhile the plants would survive in pots in the garden of the Dutch House. Alistair found a self-seeded beech sapling growing among the rhododendrons, about three-foot tall, and dug that up. They showed us a seventeen-year-old beech tree growing in the paddock, so that we knew what to expect. To this they added cuttings of the honeysuckle, Virginia creeper and wisteria. Because we were travelling by train, there was a limit to what we could take with us. We loaded it into the boot of Bernard's car, and he drove us to Kildare Station for the 19:16 train. We stood on the edge of the platform, surrounded by greenery; a portable arboretum, said Aidan, as the train drew to a stop. When we had settled ourselves in an almost empty carriage the guard came and told us that this train did not normally stop at Kildare, but the driver was so intrigued by the couple with the big clump of greenery on the platform that he decided to oblige us. It seemed like a very good omen.

That perfect day at Springfield explained a lot about Aidan to me, including his obsession with his birthplace and the childhood years that he had spent there. He was thirteen when his father Bart finally admitted defeat.

He woke his wife Lil in the night in tears to tell her 'It's all gone, Lil, it's all gone'; 'it' being the money he had inherited from a wealthy Higgins uncle in California. Bart was nominally a racehorse trainer, but according to Aidan he did little or no work beyond scuffling the gravel at the front of the house. He gave his sons a perfect 'big house' childhood, unusual for a Catholic family, and sent them to the Jesuits at Clongowes to be educated. They grew up with the assumption that life would always be like this, only to have it taken away from them, and to be sent forever into exile. No longer would he and Lil drive up to stay at the Shelbourne for the Horse Show, or the Great Southern for the Galway Races. In 1941 the family moved to an uncomfortable bungalow in Greystones where Lil, who had always had at least two servants, would have to manage without 'help'. Aidan and Colman were allowed to stay on at Clongowes at a reduced rate. The eldest son, Desmond, who was studying to be a chartered surveyor, had a mental breakdown soon after leaving Springfield, and spent some months in an institution. Brendan left for London and a clerical job at the British Film Institute. He returned to stay with a friend in Chapelizod for two weeks every summer, travelling to Celbridge daily and walking the perimeter of his former home. He lived in 'digs' all his life, working at the same job until retirement. Only the youngest son, Colman, seems to have escaped the spell of Springfield. He became an architect with a strong modernist aesthetic, having worked with the Russian architect Berthold Lubetkin after qualifying. He was interested in utopian villages and small, efficient houses. The modest home he eventually built for himself and his wife in the wild Wicklow countryside was as far removed from the traditional charm of Springfield as possible.

The memory of our visit is like a cameo in time, a beautiful place, existing outside the normal everyday. The obsession with Springfield was fully revealed and understood.

*

About a year before I met Aidan, a friend who had been the Kinsale Correspondent for the *Irish Examiner* – doing court reporting and other bits and pieces – decided to leave Kinsale.

'Why don't you take on the job?' she asked. 'It's dead easy, and you're a member of the NUJ.'

So I was, but I was a writer, not a reporter. The money was terrible, but I liked the idea of attending the monthly sitting of the Urban District Court, and learning more about the place where I was now living, seeing the community from the inside. And it would be a change to do something that didn't involve reading a book, that got me out into the world. I would also have to report on the meetings of the Kinsale Urban District Council, and anything newsworthy that happened – the opening of a new ice plant for the fishermen or the arrival of a new rector. The job was paid by the column inch, which was some compensation for intermittent tedium. So I contacted the newsroom at the *Examiner* (known locally as 'the paper', as if there was only one), who were delighted to have a volunteer with the right 'qualifications' (union membership), and I got my instructions. These were to ask the man from the *Southern Star*, Leo McMahon, to explain court reporting to me. Leo was a few years younger than me, and also had an English accent, as his parents had emigrated from Cork when he was a child. He was devoted to local reporting, and loved his job as Cork City correspondent at the *Southern Star*, incorporating the *Skibbereen Eagle*. This *Skibbereen Eagle* was famous for its international outlook, and its stern editorial warning in 1898, that it would 'keep its eye on the Emperor of Russia, and all such despotic enemies of human progression'.

Leo and I were not competitors, but rather complementary. I was working for a national daily, and Leo for a local weekly. He immediately briefed me on the pitfalls of court reporting. The chief thing was to be sure to have the correct name and address for the people up before the court: always copy it directly from the charge sheet held by the Clerk of the Court: accept no other source. Even the solicitors sometimes made mistakes in their paperwork. There might be more than one person called John Daly or Mary Kelly, so I had to have the correct address for the person before the court, otherwise the John or Mary at the wrong address would sue for defamation, and I would be out of a job.

Aidan was amazed to see the Great Patrician Scholar getting up early and dressing in an outfit that would pass for professional. It was the first Thursday in December, court day in Kinsale, and the town was buzzing with both uniformed and plain-clothes gardaí, unmarked and fully marked squad cars, and large saloons belonging to the solicitors. The Justices of the Peace, recruited from the ranks of senior solicitors to preside over the court, were usually strong characters who often enlivened the proceedings by sharp comments and dry wit. My favourite, Justice Brendan Wallace, nearly always greeted the accused by barking the order 'Take your hands out of your pockets when addressing the court.' He once remarked wearily to a fisherman denying his use of monofilament nets that fishermen had been known as liars ever since St Peter. Aidan greatly enjoyed my account of the day in court, and sometimes sat in the public gallery for an hour or so.

Between the District Court and the Council meetings, the range of people I knew in Kinsale widened considerably. My Irish family were not from the town itself, but from Summercove, a village two kilometres from the town. This makes a big difference in a small place. My grandfather and his father before him were in the Munster Fusiliers, stationed at Charles Fort, so were definitely not Kinsale townspeople, neither merchants nor professionals. Garrison folk was the old description.

It was a big change for me, moving from Summercove into the Dutch House in the centre of Kinsale, and getting to know the various corners of this half-run-down, partly done-up old town. The streets were potholed and sometimes muddy, there were vacant lots and crumbling stone walls at every turn. Some houses lacked roofs, and the gutters of the larger Georgian houses swung precariously, half-detached, after every gale, until someone pulled them off. The first time I did the famous 360-degree walk around Compass Hill I thought I had come to another village when I reached the modest terraced houses of Ballinacubby, until I spotted the tower of St Multose Church, and realised I was at the east side of the centre of Kinsale. I had walked around the hill above the town in a circle and come back in.

*

In 1987 *The Joy of Sex*, Alex Comfort's how-to manual, had just been banned for the second time in Ireland. Contraception was still illegal. It was a far cry from the swinging city (London) where I had left school some twenty-one years before. Stan, who was frequently in London, kindly collected my pills for me at the Margaret Pyke Centre in Soho every three months, and brought them back in his luggage. In return I gave him lifts to and from the airport. When I was in London I usually brought back a copy of *Playboy* magazine, also banned in Ireland, for the mechanic who kept my car on the road. Aidan referred to him ever after as 'the Ballinspittle pornographer'.

Aidan wrote a wonderful description of the frustrations of heavy petting in the opening sequence of *Dog Days*, an experience which was typical of his generation. He did not have full sex until he left Ireland for England in his mid-twenties, and met the liberal-minded South African Jill Anders, who was to become his wife.

I first had sex at the age of seventeen, relatively late among my contemporaries, with Ilya, a pal whom I liked very much, who was to remain a lover for many years. We were happy to be intimate, but we were not in love with each other, and our relationship was never exclusive. I had other friends like that. Sometimes it started as a big romance, but more often it was just another form of friendship, a bit of fun. A lot of fun in fact. We had all read *The Joy of Sex*, and followed its suggestions with enthusiasm. My generation had reliable contraception, and AIDS had not yet struck.

Aidan did not ask too many questions about my past. He was not interested in casual partners, although of course he had had a few, only Great Loves. These are described in detail in *The Whole Hog*. With the exception of his wife Jill, who also started as a Great Love, his Great Loves were remarkable mainly for how little time he spent with them, compared to how much he wrote about them. The most written-about Love is the one in *Bornholm Night-Ferry*, whom he names as Nanna Jeiner. He and Nanna were writing each other passionate love letters for some six years, but only spent a total of maybe nine days and nights together in that time.

The only past lovers he questioned me closely about were Ilya, and my husband, Paco, whom I married ten days after my twenty-first birthday. Paco and I had already been together for a year in Mexico City, while I was officially on a language year as part of my degree in Latin American Studies, and we stayed together for another five years. The marriage was precipitated by the need to sort out our respective residency permits, and enable Paco to apply for a grant to study architecture in London, and was also to satisfy my mother's idea of propriety.

The memoir I wrote for Aidan about my time in Mexico City in the 1970s is a strange piece of writing that has something of the quality of a naïve painting. It started with a story called 'Stolen Miracles' that I had written in 1970. That was the year I decided to take an optional language year as part of my degree in Latin American Studies, and spend it in Mexico with Paco, supporting myself by working as a model. The original is an episodic, largely comic account of a well-brought-up young woman, Irish but educated in 'swinging' London, getting to know Paco's family, a colourful collection of bourgeois intellectuals, and learning a whole new set of domestic conventions while also mastering Spanish. The reader follows her progress in Spanish, and parts of the early chapters are in that language, in 'lesson form', so that readers can follow the action, while also improving their Spanish. I called it *Doña Pilar* after the main character, a classical guitarist, who was based on Paco's mother. In real life she was a distinguished neuropathologist who had been a Marxist in her youth, and married a handsome architect, who turned out to be a philanderer. She had barred him from the house he had built for the family in a fashionable suburb, and lived there alone in some style, presiding over a formal Saturday lunch, attended by all four of her grown-up children and their partners, usually at least a dozen around the table. Gradually my character sees through Paco's stylish but shallow façade, preferring the more considered values of his mother and siblings. In this version of the story, I part company with Paco in Mexico after finding him in flagrante with the teenage maid. I move in with his mother, give up modelling and start taking courses at the university. As in real life, I remained good friends with his mother and his siblings long after I left Mexico.

★

The differences in our age and background had no effect on our compatibility. And I discovered as I read more of Aidan's work that we shared a fondness for outdoor sex, preferably near the sea. It was not difficult to find secluded spots around Kinsale, which I knew very well, including the Old Head of Kinsale, long favoured as a late night 'courting' spot.

When Aidan was invited to give a reading at Galway Arts Centre in late July 1987, his first thought was that this would be a perfect opportunity to take me to the Aran Islands, specifically Inishere. His plan was to swim naked before having me among the rocks at the back of the island. Joy!

We did not go directly to Galway, but made a detour via Tralee, a two-hour drive, to visit my mother who was in hospital there after a bad fall in which she had fractured her pelvis. It probably happened due to a small stroke, a transient ischaemic attack, known as a TIA. I had already been to Tralee the week before, part of a family rota to keep my father company, and to sit with my mother, who was still unconscious. I was not good at hospital visiting, permanently anxious that she might come round, and need more help than I could offer. My brother was exactly the same; we once collided in our rush to get out of her room and summon help.

Pa and I stayed in the nearest B&B to the hospital, a modern house called Manor Lodge. We had gone out for a nightcap, and we talked about Aidan for the first time. My father thought Aidan and I got on well because we both tend to be silent for most of the day: 'My headmaster used to say to me when I was head boy, I like going for walks with you, Hopkin, because you don't talk the whole time.' Then he told a long story that I had never heard before about a dawn walk up Scafell with the headmaster on a walking holiday in the Lakes that was his treat for being head boy, and a 10 a.m. breakfast at an inn that served home-cured ham and pints of bitter. It reminded me of Malcolm Lowry at the same age. I had forgotten that my father had been head boy at Worcester, and also, like Aidan at Clongowes, Captain of Cricket. It was a long walk he said, and then they had to walk back again, but by a different route, and in all that time, they met no other walkers. Today, he said, the Fells would be crowded, or so he had read.

The barman was discreetly offering us an after-hours drink, and my father was impressed that I had recognised the signals. 'Are you sure Aidan really wants to settle down in Kinsale, after all that travelling?' he asked. 'Yes,' I said. I'm sure.'

★

My mother had been conscious for some days now, but it was the first day that she was able to walk, with some help. She was slow to recover, and seemed to have aged terribly. 'Pain does not suit Angela' was Aidan's comment.

My father was in low spirits, blaming himself for the accident. However, trying to sort out the logistics of getting my mother back to London, and finding her a hospital bed there, had perked him up since my last visit. It always seemed to be raining in Tralee in those days, even though it was July, and it was drizzling once again when we drove up to the hospital. Afterwards we went for a sandwich lunch at the pub nearby, the same one where my father had his evening pint. He commented disapprovingly on the proliferation of teapots and pints of milk in the pub at lunchtime. In those days many Irishmen, especially countrymen, liked a pint of milk with their lunch. Aidan solemnly agreed it was a terrible sight, but praised the lack of background music. Aidan made considerable efforts to entertain Pa, telling him about our planned trip to Inishere.

Galway was another two hours or so further on. We took the car ferry across the River Shannon to County Clare, where we noticed with pleasure a signpost to Labasheeda – Bed of Silk – the title of a poem by Nuala Ní Dhomhnaill. As soon as we reached the County Clare side of the estuary, the rain stopped, as Aidan observed.

Aidan was always a model passenger. As a non-driver he had worked out long ago that the duty of the passenger was to keep the driver alert with amusing conversation, and by suggesting frequent stops for refreshments. I was curious about a horse fair in the streets of Kilrush, so we made a stop there, and picked our way past the horses and donkeys tethered on the pavement, in between pens of sheep, to find a bar that served tea. Unlike urban Tralee at lunchtime, teapots did not proliferate in the more rustic bars of Kilrush. We also found a phone from which to ring Derek Howard, the director of the Galway Arts Centre, who had organised the reading.

We arranged to meet in a bar in Eyre Square. Derek Howard was a pleasant man, late thirties maybe, and had lived for fifteen years in England and France. He told us that he'd come back for a short visit four years before, and had been there ever since. 'Galway is a dangerous city,' he said, which alarmed me, then I realised he meant it as a compliment: 'Some people call it "the graveyard of ambition".' Aidan asked politely if he could find a bar that had neither piped music nor TV, and we moved to Tigh Neachtain's (pronounced 'Noctan's') on Cross Street, a low-ceilinged warren of snugs that Derek told us was popular with arty young people. There we joined several of his friends, including his colleague at the Arts Centre, James Harrold, all of whom seemed to make lively gesticulations as they talked, often in order to make themselves understood above the hubbub. For the first time I was introduced as Alannah Higgins. It sounded odd, like Hopkin gone wrong, but I enjoyed the strangeness. I was made to feel very welcome, interesting in myself, not merely as Aidan's companion. Unusually, I was finding it hard to hear what people were saying. I remarked on the noise level, which was much higher than in a similar Cork bar. Several male voices roared an explanation: 'It's because Galway women shout!'

They were all admirers of *Balcony of Europe*, though none of them had read *Bornholm Night-Ferry*, which had been published only four years previously. Someone had produced posters, and photocopied flyers with a caricature of Aidan, based on one of his own drawings. They were politely amazed at how much he had changed

– bigger beard, longer hair, glasses. The posters were up, and flyers for the next day's reading would be distributed around the bars later that evening, as if Galway City were a university campus.

We had a good meal upstairs at Neachtain's with Derek, then he walked us the short distance to our B&B on the waterfront below the Spanish Arch. I was amazed to see at least fifty swans gliding past on the Corrib, so I stopped to stare, remarking on their number to Derek. 'More like two hundred,' he said. I took another look, and he was right. It was an unforgettable sight, the huge flock of graceful birds sailing by in the dusk on the black, peaty waters of the river.

The B&B was a small terraced house on the water's edge, belonging to one of the Arts Centre committee members. Derek explained that it was not a commercial B&B, it was an artistic B&B. 'Does that mean we get an artistic breakfast?' asked Aidan. 'Pink grapefruit and Hennessy brandy perhaps?'

The one thing Aidan wanted after a long day on the road was a hot bath. Our room, on the first floor, was probably the biggest in the house, but seemed very small. The bathroom was a kind of annexe, accessed by opening the door of a closet containing a nest of pink nylon frillies. Hardly had Aidan sunk into the perfumed water when our hostess burst into the room shouting at the top of her voice about drips in the dining room below. Aidan and I were both dumbstruck, as she leant into the bath and pulled the plug to prevent water going into the overflow. She stayed overlong in the eerie silence that followed her rant, staring curiously at Aidan's floating member, which he liked to refer to, after Joyce, as 'the limp father of thousands'.

Over breakfast (the usual cereal and fry, alas) our kind hostess apologised for the night before and explained that the over-full bath was leaking onto some paintings in the room below that didn't belong to her, and she had overreacted without thinking. Peace was declared.

We met Derek again that morning in Neachtain's for a quick drink before the event. Galway was ahead of the rest of Ireland at that time in having a lively Arts Centre with an exhibition space that hosted readings as well as other events in an old building on Nun's Island in the city centre. Like most other places in Galway, so it seemed, it was not far from Neachtain's. This was a lunchtime reading, and it started to drizzle as we walked from Neachtain's to the venue. 'Good for bringing a crowd in,' said Derek.

The room was brightly lit with high windows, large and stark. This was the first time I would hear Aidan reading in public, and in spite of the friendly welcome the night before, I was extremely nervous for his sake. The reading started fifteen minutes late, with an audience of about thirty, at least half of whom were either working at the Arts Centre or on its committee. I sat at the far corner of the first row, frozen with nerves and tension. Aidan found it hard to judge the volume of his voice between the microphone and the echo, and delivered an improvised chat, a series of non sequiturs in fact, while he warmed up. He had chosen 'Helsingør Station', a story from an as yet unpublished collection. It was eighteen pages long, and written largely in the second person, addressing his Danish girlfriend – the one who featured in *Bornholm Night-Ferry*. There were many good lines in it, and memorable images. But the intimacy of its tone, the change of voice from male narrator to female participant, made it an awkward piece to read aloud in broad daylight in a stark hall in drizzly Galway. As is often the case with Aidan's work, it was hard to follow chronologically. He had been reading in that inflectionless, detached voice for about forty-five minutes. Several people had left discreetly, tiptoeing out on the creaking wooden floorboards. Aidan continued, describing an amorous encounter outside the house of the polar explorer Knud Rasmussen – 'Before entering these hallowed precincts I enter you near the cliff-face in the long grass, removing the minimum of clothes. We hear Danish voices passing amicably through the hidden paths.'

Already the reading seems far too long. Everyone is shifting on the hard wooden chairs. Suddenly the reader stops, and puts down his script. 'I must be boring you, droning on. Enough of this rubbish! Any questions?'

'Why do you write rubbish?' From a young man with a German accent.

Aidan, quick as a flash, 'I was only being modest. I think it's superb.' Laughter and applause.

There are ten pages, the second half of the story, unread. He should have edited it, bearing in mind that people would be hearing it for the first time. It was misjudged, and gave the impression of being ill-prepared, which was far from the case. He had been planning this reading for weeks.

But even so, hearing the story read in the author's own voice, once he had lost his initial self-consciousness, was a very interesting experience. Derek and the other Arts Centre people were well pleased with the event. The all-important cheque, which was to fund our trip to Inishere, was handed over. Aidan was very dissatisfied with the occasion, and blamed the microphone, the acoustics and the time of day. He vowed never to give another reading, ever.

Meanwhile there was more shouting in Neachtain's with the Arts Centre people. On hearing of our plans to travel to Inishere, a woman who had lived there for a while talked non-stop about the island. There were ghosts in the abandoned coastguard house where one of the keepers fishing from a rock had been swept away by a rogue wave. Don't walk that way in the dark. Her cat killed itself on Inishere by walking into the sea because it didn't speak Irish.

I had been told that people were different in the west, but this was not what I had expected.

I was tempted by some home-made pizza and lasagne on display at the bar, but Aidan assured me we would be fed handsomely later in the O'Toole's bar in Bealadangan. We walked down the street, busy with Saturday shoppers, to pay a courtesy visit to Madame Kenny of Kenny's Bookshop. It was just as well we called by, because he was expected. Aidan was greeted like a long-lost son. The Kennys had of course heard about the reading, and his photograph was hung in a prominent place near Madame Kenny's 'pulpit'. Over the years the Kennys had photographed just about every writer in Ireland, and the black-and-white portraits lined the walls of the three-storey shop. I was duly posed and photographed to add to the archive.

For several months one winter Aidan had lived nearby at Bealadangan, beside the causeway that connected a series of islands – Annavaughan, Gorumna and Lettermore – to the mainland. It was 1977, and he had been given a grant by the American-Irish Foundation (later the Ireland Fund) to spend time back in his native land and write about it. Visits to Galway City, especially Kenny's Bookshop, were a frequent escape from the cold and isolation of the damp holiday home he was living in at the time, one of a cluster of four 'traditional' thatched cottages newly built for the tourist trade.

The heavy mist or drizzle had turned into solid rain by the time we set out on the coast road to Bealadangan. Beyond the honky-tonk plastic signage of Galway's seaside suburb, Salthill, the coast was dotted with one-off modern bungalows, each standing forlorn in its own field, in between untended scrubland.

This is his description of his time at Bealadangan from *The Whole Hog.* He got the date wrong in the published book. I have corrected it from 1985 to 1977. He was sharing the cottage with a Dublin writer and journalist, Rosita Sweetman:

> It was a thatched cottage in a group of four or five, later torched by one of the local disgruntled lads who had been refused employment by our kindly landlord Johnny O'Toole, owner of the cottages and landlord of An Hooker pub opposite, where he slept with his wife Lucy and a shotgun for protection. Against arson and grudges of course he had no protection, in a remote place where grudges were assiduosly cultivated.
>
> We drove to Galway town in her green Ford for provisions, washing, Gauloises and spirits, and it rained for six weeks without stopping. The old postman came cycling over the causeway to deliver damp parcels of books, with a permanent drip depending from the tip of his old discoloured nose and I offered him morning shots of Jameson, fearing he would otherwise never make it back to the PO.[4]

In August 1987, the burnt-out cottages had been open to the elements, and untouched since the fire some ten years earlier. The baths were covered in slime, the upstairs room, where Aidan had worked, was open to the elements. Nothing had been cleared up; the fire could have happened only days earlier.

The O'Tooles were pleased to see Aidan, and seemed genuinely fond of him. Lucy greeted Aidan as Mr Higgins, and was immediately corrected. Sandwiches had been prepared, tea (for the driver) and hot whiskey were supplied, but it was clear Aidan found their physical decline very sad to see. Johnny was wearing dark glasses, and suffering from a brain tumour that caused trembling and double-vision. Lucy was waiting for a hip replacement, and Aidan told me she had aged greatly in ten years. Neither of them were able to do much around the place. Unusually for Aidan, the conversation faltered and faded out once initial greetings had been exchanged. They kindly cashed the reading cheque – £85 – which was to pay for our stay in Inishere. We did not stay long. 'A shadow of their former selves,' was Aidan's comment.

Our next destination, the studio of the sculptor Eddie Delaney, near Carraroe, was only a few miles away. Carraroe, in turn, was just across the sound from Rossaveale, where we were to get the ferry to Inishere the next morning. We hesitated, as everyone we had met in Galway seemed to have a story about Eddie's bad behaviour, even the enfeebled Johnny O'Toole, who came briefly to life describing Eddie creating a disturbance in a new Breton restaurant that had opened nearby. I feared we were about to meet another Desmond O'Grady. I had seldom seen Aidan hesitate, but he did. He rang Bob Quinn, an artist and film-maker who lived nearby, but there was no reply. So Aidan somewhat reluctantly rang Delaney, as he called him, and we arranged to meet in the newly built Hotel Carraroe. The only shiny new building in the village, the hotel would be easy to find.

It was just as well we made contact, because we were expected, and we spent an enjoyable night with Aidan's old friend Eddie, his young partner Dr Annie Gillan and several inquisitive children who came and went like wild things.

The hotel lounge on a Saturday late afternoon was swarming with wedding guests in their finery, most of them much the worse for drink. (Was everyone in Connemara drunk all the time, or only on Saturday afternoons?) The famous Delaney, a large man in mud-splattered green wellies and an equally muddy waxed greatcoat, followed by several small, muddy children, walked in as if he owned the place. I recognised at once that he was one of those larger-than-life characters whom people either love or hate. The shouting women of Galway hated him, called him rude and brazen, but I liked him on sight, and his family, which ranged from toddlers to older children from his first marriage on a visit.

Eddie took us back to his house, a large open-plan space on two levels that he called the *atelier*. Large plate-glass windows overlooked the sea, with pots of bright red geraniums on the floor in front of them. We all left our boots at the door, and spent the evening in socks, after drying ourselves in the inglenook of an enormous log fire. We ate with the children at a long refectory table. Eddie was an enthusiastic talker, known for his malapropisms. On meeting Princess Margaret, he had remembered to call her ma'am, but had come out with 'You're looking rodent, ma'am'. He was now one of Ireland's leading artists. Having learnt all that he could in Dublin at the National College of Art and Design, without actually enrolling, as he couldn't afford to, he had continued his studies in Rome and Munich. He and Aidan had been on the fringes of Dublin's arts scene at the same time in the late 1940s. He had major public works in Dublin, including his statue of Wolfe Tone, and the Famine Memorial on St Stephen's Green. These had caused much controversy back in the mid-1960s, being the first full-scale metal sculptures most people had seen in an expressionistic idiom, and he had defended his work eloquently against its detractors.

Annie had cooked a pair of chickens for us, and we had brought wine from Galway, but in the course of an extended meal we ran out of drink. Annie and I made a foray to the nearest bar, a smoke-filled rustic den packed to the rafters with red-faced Irish-speaking men, for more vodka. 'They'll serve her, because she's the doctor,' Eddie explained. 'But they wouldn't sell me anything at this hour of the night.' Sure enough, the sea of humanity parted to let 'Doctor Annie' through to the counter, just minutes before closing time. We each bought a naggin, the only available measure. At the end of the evening, Aidan unusually gave Annie a big hug. Like me, he had felt entirely at home with the Delaneys.

There was a field beyond the house containing large metal sculptures by Eddie that I very much wanted to see, but we didn't have time to negotiate the muddy paths before catching the ferry. We could see the field clearly from the boat, however, and a line of children standing on a ditch, waving at us enthusiastically in front of a giant metal sunflower. As we sailed by, the sun came out.

This was Aidan's fourth visit to Inishere, the smallest of the three Aran islands, and my first. Distracted by the Galway reading and my mother's hospital stay, neither of us had noticed that it was the August bank holiday weekend, the height of the Irish summer. We had nothing booked, and could have been badly stuck. But strangely the island didn't seem to be unusually busy. The skipper of the *Dun Aengus* pointed us to a B&B when we docked at the pier, and the woman of the house had a room for us. It turned out he was her nephew. An old man sat in the front garden, silent, twisting wet sally rods into traditional baskets. A comatose sheepdog lay across the threshold, and the door opened to a gentle push. As Aidan had told me, there were no keys on

Inishere. We dropped our bags with the *bean an tí*, I changed into shorts, and we headed for a nearby building labelled 'Restaurant'. A young woman met us at the door and apologised: they had forgotten to put on the spuds, could we come back in half an hour?

One of the first books that Aidan had given me was J. M. Synge's *The Aran Islands*, but it had not prepared me for the physical beauty of the place. We walked up towards the air strip and back again across the sandy beach as we waited for the spuds. I was entranced; the lack of cars produced an unusually deep silence, and the birdsong rang out sharply. The colours seemed muted: pale sand, flat land covered in grey stone everywhere you looked, small whitewashed houses, pale-blue sea and sky, meeting on the far horizon. Every tiny stone-walled field held a wealth of meadow grasses and wild flowers – harebells, scabious, ox-eye daisies, saxifrage, bloody cranesbill, and samphire clinging to the rocks.

The same young one waited on our table. 'Is the soup home-made?' I asked, having glimpsed a bowl being served at another table. She went off to the kitchen to ask, and came back to say, 'No, it's from a packet.' Such honesty.

The walk we took that afternoon to the back of the island was probably unchanged since Aidan's visit in 1956, before his two-year journey around Africa with the puppets. He described it in *Balcony of Europe*: 'We walked around Inishere one afternoon, by the lake, the tall lighthouse, the long rusted hulk gone aground on the rocks (a cargo of Vat 69), kelp, rocks, wreck, a rabbit or two, gulls: all progress, all human history, was reduced to that.'[5]

We both planned to write about Inishere. Aidan had written to the new editor of the *Irish Times* proposing a piece on the changes since his previous visits nearly twenty years earlier. He hadn't had a reply, but that didn't seem to bother him. I wondered why he hadn't written to the features or travel editor, but said nothing. I thought that perhaps when you were as well established as he was, you went straight to the top. It never occurred to me that I could have helped him with my more professional approach, and advised him to contact the features editor, Caroline Walsh, who later, once the strange request had eventually landed on her desk, replied saying she would have loved such a piece, but it was now too late in the season.

I was planning a travel piece, probably for *The Guardian*, which had used my work before, but didn't query anyone in advance, as I didn't need to think about expenses. I spent much of my time on the island writing compulsively in a dedicated notebook, combining personal impressions with Aidan's stories of the old days, and facts gleaned from various tourist booklets and a book I had bought in Kenny's of Galway, *A World of Stone: Life, Folklore and Legends of the Aran Islands*. 'Limestone paving: Clints: the blocks that constitute the paving, Grykes: open crevices isolating individual clints. The size and shapes of the clints depends on the frequency of the grykes.' I loved these strange new words. Aidan noted them mentally for future use in Scrabble, and commented: 'When you fear for your cyst think of your fistula. And when you tremble for your fistula, consider your chancre.' He did not appear to take any notes about the island at all. As far as I know, he never wrote up our trip.

Instead of the ubiquitous morning fry, we were offered a fresh mackerel fillet, lightly fried and served with home-baked soda bread. Our landlady let us take the remains of the bread for our lunch, which we supplemented with a block of bright orange Galtee cheese, and apples from the island's only shop. Then we walked an hour or so to the back of the island, where we skinny-dipped and napped, and found a storm wall of three-metre-high boulders among which we could do whatever we liked unobserved by anyone else. We sat in the shelter of the rusted hulk to eat our picnic and talk: we were still getting to know each other, and it was good to be alone, away from Kinsale and the daily routine. By early evening we were back at the B&B, setting up the Scrabble board. Sometimes we had another swim after the game, from the sandy beach nearby. Aidan was a good strong swimmer, with a relaxed front crawl that looked as if he could go on for ever.

There were not many other people about, and the main entertainment consisted in observing a pack of dogs of various shapes and sizes, waiting their turn to mate with a small spaniel bitch that was on heat. When we walked among the stone-walled fields near our B&B we saw an old man in a bawneen sweater carrying a plastic bucket on his way to milk his cow. Because the fields were so small, there was only room for one cow in each. They looked sulky and bad-tempered. 'Cows are herd animals,' Aidan said. 'They need company.' That made sense: I was impressed at his countryman's knowledge. With his cosmopolitan background it was easy to forget that he had had what he called 'a rustic upbringing'.

In the evening we had a choice of a simple meal at the hotel (steak or chops or fish) with a red candle on the table, or the restaurant (roast meat, vegetables and boiled potatoes) followed by a couple of nightcaps in one of the island's three pubs. The quiet, mannerly men that Aidan remembered drinking in the bars thirty years before had been replaced by rowdy youngsters and much drunkenness, perhaps because of the bank holiday, which featured a highly competitive rowing regatta. Thomas O'Flaherty, the father of today's barman, had once refused Aidan a third gin and tonic; he considered two such drinks to be enough for anyone. Another time Aidan had to wait while the family rosary was concluded in the kitchen before he could be served a drink. He remembered that they had said Thomas O'Flaherty should have been a bishop. His son laughed at the memory, and bought us both a drink.

But his contemporaries did not all share this attitude. We witnessed an unpleasant scene the next evening in another bar run by a young man called Piaras. A frail and elderly American woman in dark glasses made her way up to the bar around 5 p.m. in a state of high anxiety to ask about the ferry back to the mainland:

'Has the last ferry left? They say the ferry went at four thirty but we were told on the way over that it was going back at six thirty.' She had a flat American accent.

Piaras and his contemporaries up at the bar exchanged bored glances. One man said something in Irish and another answered him in an interrogative tone. Piaras was polishing a glass.

'Is there another ferry to Doolin today?' She was paler now, trembling slightly and biting her lip. 'Does anyone know if there's another Doolin ferry?'

They all looked at Piaras.

'I don't know the ferry times,' he said, still polishing the glass. 'Ask them below at the pier.'

That was obviously where she had just come from.

She turned and fled.

This was the sort of churlish behaviour that Aidan abhorred, but he knew better than to say so to a group of young island men. Rather than making him angry, it saddened him, which was somehow worse. It signified the end of a kinder era.

The details of Aidan's earlier trips to Inishere are vague; it seems Colman was there too, and their mother, so perhaps they were very young. Then when he met Jill, his future wife, he decided he had to show her this extraordinary place. He worked extra shifts in the cold room at the Wall's Ice Cream Factory near Willesden Junction to save enough money for the journey from London. When they reached Inishere on a fine day in August, among the first people they met were Colman and his wife Sylvia. His friend John Beckett was also there, with his girlfriend Vera Slocum.

'Didn't you find that strange?' I asked. 'All these people you knew just happening to be on Inishere at the same time?'

'No.'

Then one evening, our fifth, we realised we'd had enough of Inishere, enough fried mackerel and soda bread, enough rocky paths, fornicating dogs and lonely cows, and told our landlady we'd be leaving in the morning. Our bill for the B&B came to £75, just within budget. As we left, we bought a large turf basket woven from sally rods from the man working away in the front garden, a handsome piece of work that we used as a log basket for many years.

I had been working hard on the notes I had taken on Inishere. It was not working out as a travel piece – partly because I had not gone alone, partly because an honest description of the island would have had to include the rudeness and drunkenness we had witnessed, and that would not have been acceptable for the holiday market. But I could see the Inishere piece as a short story, and that was much more interesting. But before writing either, I was dutifully typing up all the notes from the two notebooks I had been keeping – my regular daily diary and a special travel notebook – as I had been advised to do by Ernest Gébler: 'No short cuts, never take short cuts with your writing.'

After an unusually boozy dinner with Derek Mahon, who had discovered after seven years on the dry, that he could, as he put it, 'take the occasional drink', when we got home, Aidan let slip that he had been reading 'my Inishere stuff' and did not think much of it. The notes were dead, I'd been looking at the wrong things. I was outraged. How dare he read my diary and my private notebook, when I had specifically asked him not to? He looked sheepish, which he did very well. Instead of hitting him, as he deserved, I burst into tears. I thought I caught a look of satisfaction, a small smirk at the spectacle – his little devil playing up again. So as quickly as I had started, I stopped crying, went to the bathroom to wash my face, and straight to bed.

Once I lay down, I started to see the funny side of it: if he had liked what he read, I wouldn't have minded him reading it at all. It was only him not liking it that had upset me. To hell with what he thinks. I resolved to continue with my typing, work damn hard at it, and prove him wrong. The resulting story, 'The Dogs of Inishere', was eventually published in the USA and in *Books Ireland*, and became the title story of my first collection.

★

My birthday, 6 September 1987
Present from Aidan:
The Islandman by Tomás O'Crohan
The Poor Mouth by Flann O'Brien
The Boarding House by William Trevor
If Not Now, When? by Primo Levi

★

We could not go on for ever, shifting from the small apartment to the bigger house by the sea and back. The obvious next move was to buy a house together. I was pleased that Aidan took me seriously enough to consider this major step. After the initial conversation about buying a house, we didn't mention the matter again for about six months, and when we did, I was incredulous. No words of love had been exchanged after the intitial agreement that they were superfluous, but we had had many minor 'spats', mostly about literary matters, and often fuelled by late-night drinking. There had also been complaints from him about my late nights 'carousing' (one of Aidan's favourite words) with friends, chiefly because I usually woke him up on coming home.

For my part, I was often annoyed at his unpredictable daytime disappeareances: while he was usually home by six for Scrabble, some days he lost track of time, and didn't appear until 8 or 9 o'clock, well after our usual supper time, leaving me unsure whether to eat or wait. The first time he stayed out all night, smoking and tippling with our neighbour Stan, I was worried he'd come to some harm. He also had a habit of leaving whatever company we were in if he got bored, and not bothering to tell me he was going home – he had 'vapourised', as we called it. So I was often left doing a round of cafés or pubs looking for Aidan, while he was already safely at home. It especially annoyed me when he did this at other people's houses, because it was bad manners, and I didn't hesitate to tell him so. We were by no means the perfect couple. Suddenly I needed reassurance. I had to ask, 'Are you really sure you want to buy a house with me?' to which he answered with some surprise and not a moment's hestitation, 'Yes, of course'.

He later told me that the moment when he had known I was the right woman for him had been my tact, as he called it, while we drove Carl and Carlota home from the bus station, my staying silent and not intruding on his reunion with his son, thereby making it easier for all concerned. It had seemed to me only the natural thing to do.

As a deposit Aidan offered the savings – around £4,000 – he had acquired while teaching Creative Writing ('a trade recondite as falconry') at the University of Texas in Austin. I had no savings to speak of, in spite of having optimistically opened an account with the Educational Building Society a few years before. The remaining St Patrick money would pay off my overdraft and put me back in the black, but there would not be much left over. But being younger, and officially self-employed, with annual accounts to prove it, I should manage to qualify for a mortgage. Our very own bank, the AIB, was plastered with posters advertising mortgages, which banks had only recently starting offering. Before that you had to build up savings with a specialised 'Building Society' to qualify. We were friendly with our bank manager, and often had a drink with him in the Armada, so we reckoned our prospects were good.

We had our eye on the house next door to my parents' house on the quay at Summercove, an old three-storey, semi-detached building with an ominous-looking crack in its gable end, and a slightly impeded sea view, both of which made it affordable. It faced southwest, and had a bright, sunny first-floor sitting room. It was owned by a local builder. He offered it to us for £17,000. He would fix the gable end for us himself. Once that was done all it needed was partial rewiring and new bow windows. We explained this to our friendly bank manager, then went back a few weeks later and sat beneath the advertisement for mortgages while we were given a straightforward no. Our bank manager explained that much as he would like to oblige us, the mortgage department would not lend money to two self-employed people, one of whom had no annual accounts and two overdrafts, for a house they considered uninhabitable.

Aidan often teased me about my devotion to the reading of local newspapers, but it was because of this habit that I discovered a new County Council scheme to enable people on low incomes to buy their first house. I did some sums, and realised that I would qualify. With Aidan's savings as a deposit, and a County Council mortgage in my name, we could do it, even though the title deeds would have to be in my name only. That could be sorted out later. All we needed now was to find a house within our budget. We went to the local auctioneer, Denis Sheehy of Sheehy Brothers. There were two possibilities: a gloomy, square-built 1950s' bungalow on the edge of town, surrounded by huge leylandii, or a small old terraced house in the centre of town with a long back garden, the width of two houses. 'You'd be getting a bargain there,' said Denis Sheehy, 'The owner reduced it by £3,000 only this morning to get it off his hands before the winter.'

The bungalow was not possible, we were both so oppressed by the tall dark trees, which would cost a lot of money to remove, that we hardly looked at the house, beyond noting it was small, dark and damp. The stone-built little house at the bottom of a hill in the medieval town centre had been empty for some time, and was being used to store apples from its garden. Its owner, a tall Englishman about my age, was fixing the front door lock when we called by to view, but did not seem inclined to chat. He had had a series of difficult tenants, he said, and was fed up with being a landlord. Aidan tried to get more information from him, and succeeded: he had moved out of the house reluctantly two years before, soon after the birth of his second child. He needed a bigger house, and found one in the country. As prices were rock-bottom, he had held on to this one as long as he could, but did not want to leave it empty for another winter. So he had reduced its price that very morning, thus putting it within our range. 'It's a perfectly good house, you'd be getting a bargain,' he said. Beyond that, he made no attempt to sell it to us, and didn't even stop to show us around. Once he had fixed the front door, he disappeared without saying goodbye.

The stone walls of the house were two feet thick, and there was no sign of damp. It had two small rooms on the ground floor, each with a sash window, and there was a bathroom extension to the rear. The top floor had been converted into one large, high-ceilinged room with exposed roof beams, a wood-burning stove, a galley kitchen and a door that led across a bridge of wooden decking to the garden, which was on the same level as the first floor of the house. It was what some locals called 'an upside-down house', with kitchen and sitting room upstairs, and bedrooms on the ground floor, a fairly common arrangement in houses with a sea view. This house had only a garden view; the street side overlooked the flat roof of an extension that had been built on to a large pub. The ground floor was dark, partly because of the decking that had been built over the back yard. I immediately claimed the small front room as my workroom. Aidan said he would like a big desk in the upstairs room.

The whole house reeked of the apples that were stored there, with overtones of rubber-backed carpet. The garden, or was it an orchard, consisted of about a third of an acre, 240 feet by 40 (73m x 12m), according to the auctioneer's brochure. It had ancient apple trees between tall grey stone walls, some of which were crumbling. It was so overgrown that you couldn't see where it ended. The square tower of St Multose Church was visible beyond the stone wall. We poked our heads over, and saw its graveyard. 'At least we'll have quiet neighbours,' said Aidan. The walled garden was the deciding factor: such space and privacy in the centre of town was a rare find. Given a year or two, it could be really beautiful. The drawbacks – a dark ground floor, no off-street parking, no guest bedroom / second study, and possible late-night noise from the pub – were all things we could live with. I liked the house for its modest scale and quiet location. While there was scope to build on at the back when we had money, it would not need much spent on it, the way the house with a sea view would have done. It would be inexpensive to run and to maintain, being so small. It would be an unpretentious but pleasant and economical place to live, ideal for two writers. Keep your overheads low, as Ernest Gébler used to advise me.

We made an offer on the house in Higher Street, and it was acccepted. It would be some time before we would be able to move in, but at least we had a plan.

Meanwhile, our apartment at the Dutch House, right under the eaves, was a cosy place to snuggle up together on a stormy night. On this particular night the storm was unusually noisy, the wind swirling around our eyrie, whistling in between the windows and their frames. The whole house shook as gust after gust hit the steeply raked roof. In between the whistles and rushes of the wind, we could hear slates smash as they flew off some roof and landed on the road. The eaves creaked in the wind, and the whole roof seemed to stretch and contract above our head. Sleep was impossible.

Usually we would have found something to talk about, but we were both over-awed by the unusual strength of the storm. The power had gone earlier in the evening – even the street lights were out – so there was no point in getting up to look out of the window. We just lay there on our backs in silence in the dark.

As another strong gust struck, Aidan put his arm across my chest at an unusual angle, as if to hold me down in the bed. It was exciting, it was an adventure, but never once was I frightened: I knew that Aidan would look after me. It was not until the next morning, early, both of us still safe in bed in the pale after-storm light, that Aidan told me he had genuinely believed that the roof was about to lift off, leaving us exposed to the elements. That was why he had pinned me down. He had been afraid. I had felt no fear at all, trusting Aidan to look after me, and knowing, deep down, that roofs simply did not blow off in this part of the world.

In that, I was wrong. It was the night of 15/16 October 1987, the night of the Great Storm, when a severe depression in the Bay of Biscay produced hurricane-force winds of up to 139 kilometres per hour that battered England, Wales and southwest Ireland, killing twenty-two people and felling an estimated 15 million trees.

★

In late November I spent some time in London helping my parents. My mother never really recovered from the fall in Kerry, and her mental state was causing concern. She continued to have TIAs, and one day found herself totally lost in her nearest department store, Peter Jones. She was at the Lancôme counter, buying face cream, and suddenly she didn't know where she was. Luckily she was a regular customer, and the woman serving her knew her. She had her account card in her hand, so they sat her down and eventually made contact with my father, who came and took her home. After that, she never went out alone, and had to be locked in the flat when my father did, but he was so tactful about it that she never noticed. Now he needed to have an operation on his cataracts, so I took over while he was in hospital.

There were underlying problems, as my father suffered from glaucoma. We knew the operation might not be a success, but it had to be done. I tried very hard to be patient, kind and sympathetic with my mother, but found it very difficult. Her helplessness and forgetfulness left her in a state of constant confusion, as I discovered when I tried to show her how to make a simple vegetable soup. There was a mess of onion, potato, celery and carrot all over the kitchen, and I couldn't even stretch out a friendly hand, lighten up by making a pleasant remark, suggest a cup of tea together, make a list – no, I just froze. I was waiting for her to take charge, because she was my mother, but she wasn't able to any more. The cooking was an attempt to distract her from constantly packing and unpacking a series of small bags in case she too had to go into hospital. Unlike my sister Pixie and her daughter, who were good at jollying my mother along and making a joke of her probems, I was long-faced and over-anxious, totally out of my depth. I was definitely not cut out to be a carer. It was a relief when my father was discharged, and I was able to go back to my life in Kinsale.

★

That Christmas was our first together. We made it a traditional one, at home alone in the Dutch House, with turkey, ham, Brussels sprouts, mashed turnip, Irish sherry trifle, home-made cake and copious good wine. Among my presents I found *If This Is a Man* by Primo Levi. I was riveted, read it in one sitting, and came to bed late. Aidan was still awake, and he told me how he first came across it in Paddy Collins' bookcase in a rented wing of Howth Castle. This was the Irish artist Patrick Collins (1910–1994), who befriended the aspiring young writer on the contrary grounds that he, Collins, wanted to be a writer, while the writer Aidan wanted to be a painter. At the time they met, Collins was still working nine to five for an insurance company in O'Connell Street, and living in Howth Castle. He was paying £12 a week, a fortune in the 1950s, and Lord Talbot de Malahide had also given Collins the right to burn any rotten timber he found in the grounds. Aidan would cycle over from Greystones for the weekend, a distance of forty-two kilometres, then spend long days sawing and hauling wood, and sleep on the sofa in front of the sitting room fire after listening all evening to Collins talk. He would often stay in on the Monday morning after Collins left for work, reading the books that his friend had been describing. This was how he discovered William Faulkner and Eudora Welty, whose books Collins had come across in the reading room of some American cultural institution off Grafton Street. Then one day Collins gave him *If This Is a Man*. At that time Aidan was very friendly with John Beckett, who also read it. John Beckett told him about seeing a copy of a new Primo Levi in the window of the Eblana Bookshop on his way to a music lesson. He went back after the lesson to buy it, and the one and only copy had been sold. Aidan said, 'You're looking at the lad who owns it.'

These were the times when Aidan lived on a shilling a day, given to him by his mother, read voraciously and travelled big distances on foot and bicycle. For a shilling you could buy an orange, a lump of Galtee cheese and a bread roll. He carried these and his books on his back in a muslin jelly bag provided by his mother. He wore corduroys that had been altered by his mother by hand, with the result that one leg was wide and the other narrow. The uppers of his shoes had parted from the soles and he had the inspired idea, it seemed to him, of tying them together with pyjama cord. He was extremely shy and never talked. Paddy Collins, on the other hand, never stopped talking, and in this way they enjoyed each other's company. Those were also the days in which he would be 'cavorting' with Arthur Power, a former art critic of the *Irish Times* who had known Joyce in Paris and who lived at Sandymount overlooking 'the beach where Bloom masturbated', in Aidan's words.

Aidan described himself in those days as a thin, silent reader, tattily dressed, riding a very good (said with emphasis) Raleigh bicycle. He was stopped by a policeman one day at the Dawson Street traffic lights, and gestured to approach him. 'I'm on to you,' said the cop with a glare. Aidan continued: 'I was half-mad in those days with malnutrition and anaemia. I ended up in Clonskeagh Fever Hospital with scarlet fever. I told the nurses there that when I got out, I was going to London to make my fortune. I told them so often that I started to believe it. So when I got out, I sold my golf clubs to a friend of my father, and took the boat to London.'

*

The sale of the house on Higher Street was only finalised on 17 December 1987, owing to complications involving a bridging loan and life insurance. But on that date, just over a year after first meeting, we were at last given the keys and became the proud owners of a house and garden.

My father's cataract operation revealed that he was also suffering from macular degeneration, and his sight, which was already limited, would be reduced to peripheral vision as the years passed. He and my mother reluctantly decided to put their house in Summercove on the market. So instead of moving to our 'winter quarters', as Aidan liked to put it, we stayed put in the Dutch House until such time as we could organise the move to the new house.

In June 1988 Aidan was invited by the Irish Arts Council to give a paper in Dún Laoghaire at the first International Writers' Conference. It was part of an Arts Council initiative to encourage the celebration of Bloomsday in Dublin, dreamt up by Lar Cassidy, the Arts Council's literature officer, and the novelist John Banville. Neither Aidan nor I had any idea of what to expect, but five nights in the Royal Marine Hotel at Dún Laoghaire sounded nice. Desmond O'Grady and Derek were invited to speak at the same event. I was invited as Aidan's partner.

Aidan had spent several weeks writing his fifteen-minute paper. We were given a large corner room at the Royal Marine, with a view of Joyce's Martello Tower in the distance. It was a blazing hot day. To recover from the journey we walked to the end of the pier and back, a daily ritual for many residents. I liked Dún Laoghaire. I always said that if I ever had to live in Dublin, that was where I would choose, and Aidan agreed.

On the way back to the hotel we took a look at Haigh Terrace, where Aidan's parents had lived very poorly towards the end of their lives. The cold basement flat in

Haigh Terrace is described so vividly in *Balcony of Europe* that I seemed to know it well:

> Flaking distemper fell from the ceiling and lay like snow, a greyish slush, on the damp linoleum that had buckled and perished here and there, by the door that would not close, under the draining-board, around the dinted and seldom disinfected bucket that had no handle, before the stove with its coating of thick grease, as Sharpe the taximan moved in the room above. He was their landlord, and the rent was low.[6]

Though the exterior had been 'tittivated up', in Aidan's words, with some fresh paint, Haigh Terrace still looked a bit sad.

There was a big crush at the Mansion House, where we were bussed for the launch of the Writers' Conference. I didn't know anybody, so I was pleased to spot Dermot Healy, in a dark suit with a pink rose in his lapel. We had met in Cootehill the previous year and had bonded instantly, perhaps through our affection for Aidan. He had not been invited to the conference, but was in Dublin for the funeral of the poet John Jordan, an old friend and mentor, who was to be buried the next day. He had heard about the conference on the grapevine, and had just come from the removal. He promised to come out to Dún Laoghaire when the funeral was over, 'to ginger things up a bit'.

Aidan introduced me to his friend John McGahern, a thin man, with a lovely gentle manner, and Nuala Ní Dhomhnaill, an Irish language poet with long red hair worn loose, and pale, almost translucent skin. Nuala in turn introduced me to Luisa Valenzuela, an Argentinean writer, who spoke the most beautiful Spanish.

Once back at the Royal Marine, we had the first of several hotel meals, described by Aidan as 'inedible'. It was just ordinary hotel fare, but he took exception to it. Nuala noticed Luisa and me talking in Spanish, and immediately insisted I should interview Luisa for the *Irish Times*. She was going to set it all up for me; it was an opportunity not to be missed. Aidan made his own circuit of the busy bar, standing back and stroking his beard while deciding whom to approach. He ended up deep in conversation with the actor Cyril Cusack, a Royal Marine regular, rather bemused at all these literary types invading his normally quiet bar. He and Aidan tackled the question of whether or not acting was an art. Aidan soon realised that Cusack was deaf in one ear, and moved to the other side, which helped Cusack to make more sense of the conversation. We both stayed talking on our separate circuits until late in the packed, overheated bar.

After breakfast we walked to the Martello Tower and the Forty Foot, in those days the male-only swimming place. As we walked back past Haigh Terrace, Aidan described coming home from South Africa via England with Jill and their son Carl, still a baby, and being met off the ferry by his father, and the taxi belonging to his parents' landlord, Sharpe. His father met the mail boat every morning when it docked at No. 2 berth shortly after seven o'clock, and watched the passengers disembark: 'Three or four times a year he would see someone he knew; it made the day for him. The habit of going there had become a ritual for him, this small indomitable man with bowed back and vague eyes and wavery talk.'[7]

Because of the hot weather, we spent a lot of time over the next few days milling about outside the hotel, escaping from its smoky, overheated rooms. Every morning three writers per session gave fifteen-minute papers which were followed by a discussion, then a break. Aidan's paper was scheduled for the Thursday – day three, Bloomsday itself – so he had plenty of time to observe the others in action.

We were having a drink with Tom Kilroy, an admirer of Aidan's work, when we were interrupted politely by another Higgins admirer. Seeing the large sack of books that he was carrying, Aidan excused himself, and took him over to a windowsill where he could spread out his books for signing. This was my first encounter with the Higgins fan, who remained surprisingly true to type over the years. They were always male, often bearded, and usually carried a large plastic bag of well-thumbed books, or in some cases a sack.

During one of those fresh-air breaks between papers, I noticed Aidan staring with fascination at a group of people talking amongst themselves. They seemed like old friends, happy to find one another in new surroundings. As I followed his gaze I gradually identified them – the poet Joseph Brodsky, born in Russia, now living in New York; Derek Walcott, originally from St Lucia in the Caribbean, and his tall, very beautiful blonde girlfriend; the large figure of the Australian poet Les Murray, in a blue-and-white-striped shirt; and the unmistakeable figure of Susan Sontag, wearing her trademark black polo neck, in spite of the heat, her thick black hair, carelessly thrown back, cut through by a streak of white. She was talking with animation to Joseph Brodsky: 'It's a Schiller poem that *everybody* knows,' she said very loudly, then she sang in perfect pitch the opening bars of the 'Ode to Joy' – which I knew only as the choral movement of Beethoven's Ninth – and she sang in German, of course.

Derek Mahon and his friend Patricia King, an American PhD student, arrived just in time for dinner, and we shared a round table with David Lodge and Craig Raine. At some point

Dermot Healy joined us. His fast-flowing talk was confounding the partially deaf Lodge, who complained, 'I can't follow what he's saying; it's not grammatical, I'm completely lost,' which only spurred Healy on to greater heights of convoluted Cavan rhetoric. It was a stellar performance.

Dermot and I went outside to smoke. Aidan had bought him a brandy. 'He must love you very much,' he said. 'I've observed him with other women, and he treats you differently.' 'It's mutual,' I said, and he gave me a hug. He promised to come back the next day to liven things up again.

On Wednesday Luisa read an interesting paper, ranging over the Mothers of the Plaza de Mayo, and their efforts to keep the memory of the 'disappeared' alive, and her own memories of her mother, who dreamt a novel, then stayed in bed for two months to write it. She remembered the laughter between her mother and Jorge Luis Borges when they were collaborating on a story, Borges saying as he left, 'That was a great day's work. We've written two whole sentences.' I envied her this literary background: how could she not be a writer?

It was a relief to learn that Aidan had arranged for us to go to dinner in nearby Shankill with the film-maker and photographer George Morrison, an old friend who was best known for his collaboration with the composer Seán Ó Riada on the documentary, *Mise Éire*. Aidan had known George since his early twenties, when they both attended Arland Ussher's Sunday 'salons', in search of wisdom. George was now married to Theodora Fitzgibbon, who was famous as the cookery writer of the *Irish Times*. As well as a break from the literary crowd, we would also be able to eat a meal without Aidan complaining that it was 'inedible'.

Theodora was of course much more than a cookery writer. I had greatly enjoyed the two volumes of her autobiography, an account of the life of a true Bohemian in Dublin, London and the south of France. While they got on well in person, Aidan had a terrible aversion to Theodora's books. He could not understand me liking them so much – I had read the autobiography twice since meeting her, and had written to her to tell her how much I liked it. Every time Aidan saw the two books, he suggested that it was time to throw them out.

George and Theodora lived in an old house in a countrified lane which had somehow survived in the suburban sprawl of Shankill. We were ushered into the garden. Theodora was on her way back from judging a cookery competition in Wexford, and would join us later. The garden was full of flowers and beautifully overgrown. George seemed to remember every scene of every film he had ever seen, and the music that went with them, which he whistled, tunelessly.

When Theodora finally arrived, about an hour later, I thought she looked tired, and older than I remembered. She was seventy-one, to George's sixty-five. She had made lovage soup, which was served cold, Vichyssoise-style. Our main course, coq au vin, had been cooked earlier that day, by the winner of the cookery competition she had judged. There were cut-glass decanters of red and white wine on the table, and rum ice cream to finish. Theodora retired after serving the ice cream.

To sober up before driving us back to the hotel, George showed a video of Luis Buñuel's masterpiece *The Discreet Charm of the Bourgeoisie*. We got back at about 3.30 p.m., and joined John Montague, Seamus Deane, Michael Longley and his wife Edna in the bar. They were in the midst of a heated discussion that had obviously been going on for some time. Aidan immediately pitched in. I listened for a while, mesmerised by the intensity of the arguments in the unfamiliar Northern accents, before retiring at around 4.30 p.m., while Aidan stayed on talking.

The next day Aidan was scheduled to give his paper immediately after the lunch break. I attended the morning session, mainly to get out of his way, and was pleased to run into Brian Fallon, who was covering the event for the *Irish Times*. Together we listened to Thomas Kilroy talking about his gratitude for the nation's release from Catholic oppression, then Susan Sontag, 'Sontagging', as Brian called it – confidently waffling on for the prescribed fifteen minutes, not one word of which either of us could remember. She had objected to being introduced as 'one of the world's leading intellectuals', saying she was first and foremost a writer, but had written half a century of essays, some of which 'hung around her neck like an albatross'. Brian, one of the best-read people I know, told me that her novel *The Benefactor* was indeed very good.

I skipped the questions, and went to see how Aidan was getting on. The Galway fiasco had left me very nervous of him speaking in public. He had been writing his paper for weeks, ever since he had been invited, but had now decided at the last minute to rewrite it, in the light of what had gone before. This he did in longhand, standing at the window of our room. I brought a gin and tonic up for him. He took it outside, and paced up and down on the lawn to avoid having to make small talk until it was time for his event.

As luck would have it, Aidan was surrounded by friends: Anthony Cronin was chairing the session, and he was seated next to Derek Mahon, who read his poem 'The Joycecentenary Ode'. It was, after all, 16 June – Bloomsday again.

Aidan made a shaky start, then the laughs started coming and he hit his stride, concluding to warm applause.

In the break that followed I met Brian in a corridor on his way out. He was delighted with Aidan's paper. In his conference report, which appeared in the *Irish Times* the next day, he wrote:

> In the afternoon, the novelist Aidan Higgins opened proceedings, and though the word 'celebratory' had been much tossed around, his tone seemed to be of unrelieved gloom. A little halting at first he warmed to his subject as he painted a picture of the modern Apocalypse – 'Our end will come with the rats, those creatures excluded from the Ark'. The media – at least the Irish media – were not spared in his address, including 'an exceedingly bland newspaper called *The Irish Times*, written almost entirely, as it sometimes seems, by Maeve Binchy', while RTÉ was equally dominated by Gay Byrne – laughter and some applause.[8]

On my way back into the conference room, a fast-moving man passed me by, in a hurry to get somewhere, leaving behind a strong smell of cigarette smoke and an aura of negativity and danger. It was a very strange experience. Later I realised this man was Joseph Brodsky. Hermione Lee's paper was next, followed by the most memorable event of the whole conference, the Nigerian novelist Chinua Achebe's indictment of colonialism in literature, cogently illustrated by examples from Joseph Conrad's novel *Heart of Darkness*. This was the paper everyone was talking about for the rest of the evening, Aidan included.

Anthony Cronin, who was also represented by the agent Reg Davis-Poynter, introduced himself to me. 'I know your work' – he had read *The Out-haul*, and liked it. I told him Reg was also acting for Aidan now. He seemed surprised that Aidan was no longer with John Calder. And he was even more surprised to hear that we had bought a house in Kinsale. I explained how we had combined Aidan's savings with my ability to borrow money on a County Council scheme, and I could see the possibility also interested him.

For dinner that evening we were taken by coach to Temple Bar in the centre of Dublin, a journey of about half an hour. After about twenty minutes the coach stopped for a lone figure, standing on the pavement, who hopped aboard. It was Seamus Heaney, who'd been waiting outside his house in Sandymount. Temple Bar was still an interesting artistic quarter in 1988, and the restaurant we were booked into was a small French place, with tables very close together. We sat with Derek and Pat, and were joined by Nuala Ní Dhomhnaill, an admirer of Aidan's work. She was married to a Turkish man, Dogan Leflef, and had lived in Turkey for several years, and mastered the language. She told Aidan she was attracted to men by their smell, an idea that fascinated him. She told us that Brodsky was hostile to women. 'What do you write with, your hair?' he had asked her.

Back at the hotel, there were more drinks. We sat with Tom Kilroy and John and Madeline McGahern. Aidan had known John since the 1970s, when both were living in Dublin. McGahern was working as a primary school teacher, and Aidan had a wife and two children and hardly any money. He asked McGahern for the loan of a fiver to get him through the weekend, and was given £100, an unheard of sum back then. John said not to worry about repaying it. He had just sold a novel (*The Dark*). We all headed upstairs to bed sometime after 2.30 a.m., and left the McGaherns, who couldn't find their room, giggling in the corridor.

While the conference itself was officially over, everyone was staying on for a group reading on the next night, Friday

17 June, at the Royal Hospital Kilmainham. Once again, the coach stopped at Sandymount to pick up the solitary figure standing by the side of the road. Seamus was to be MC for the night, introducing each writer in alphabetical order to an audience of more than 700 people in the packed Great Hall: Chinua Achebe to Liz Lochhead, then a break; then David Lodge to Derek Walcott. By now a group dynamic had developed amongst those attending the conference, and after five days this distinguished crowd of people were starting to feel like family. Seamus's introductions were short and witty, delivered with ease, as if he'd been doing this all his life.

Next morning the perky couple, who five days earlier had carried their suitcases up the hill to the Royal Marine from the train station, could hardly lift the same cases into a taxi. It took us all the way to Heuston Station, paid for by Aidan's expenses cheque, which the hotel had cashed. The driver was an archetypal Dub, a drinking companion of the recently deceased John Jordan (he had been at the funeral that week), and a friend of Benedict Kiely. A copy of Patrick Kavanagh's *Collected Poems* was stashed in his glove compartment. When Aidan commented on that, he replied, 'I never travel without it.' But he didn't ask who his passenger was, and Aidan, ever modest, did not tell him.

★

The house in Higher Street was ours, but we were still living in the Dutch House. We had made a start on Higher Street, cleared a sunny part of the garden and planted the beech sapling from Springfield. The rest of the garden was a wildlife oasis of long grass and apple trees. The house itself needed only a small sum of money spent on it before we moved in, £1,000, say, but we didn't have even that small sum. I came home from the conference to a mountain of bills. The mortgage from the County Council had been approved, but for the eight months while it was going through the process, I was paying for an expensive bridging loan every month, while Aidan continued to pay the rent of the Dutch House. Then there was house insurance, life insurance, an increasingly unviable car, and regular living expenses. Aidan still had two overdrafts. He was, if possible, even worse at managing money than I was, and far less practical. I decided that the best way out of our situation, besides finding some well-paid work, was for me to take charge of getting us into the house at Higher Street before winter set in, and making it a priority.

In addition to all these unusual expenses, we had been living way above our means ever since we'd met, we both agreed on that. We vowed to stay out of restaurants and bars until things got back to normal. The inaugural Kinsale Arts Week, which we had helped to organise, was in full swing when we got back from Dún Laoghaire, but we scarcely had the price of a drink between us. Nevertheless, we went to the reading given by Joseph Brodsky. He read intially in English, chain-smoking, as was his habit. We were in a lofty hotel function room right on the water's edge, with views of the sea in the light of the long June evening. My former housemate, Tom Rourk, who spoke Russian, stood up as the applause died down, and asked Brodsky if he would please read a poem in Russian. He agreed, and it was as if another man had taken over the podium, a far bigger man with a stronger voice and a strength of feeling so forceful that it seemed as if the whole building was levitating. That was when I realised that this was the obverse of that icy sensation that had knocked me back in a hotel corridor in Dún Laoghaire: such strength of spirit could work as strongly for good as for evil. The audience rose to its feet as one and applauded loud and long. Nobody who was there has ever forgotten it.

★

It was a good summer, by Irish standards, dry and sunny. I was working on the garden at Higher Street, with intermittent help from Aidan. My mother had given him her golf clubs, a nice gesture, and he was playing with a variety of people – Jim Edwards, who ran a bar-restaurant in Kinsale, and Jim's golfing companions, mainly men in late middle-age who also went racing together, and occasionally my father. My father had never had the time to improve his golf handicap, and he enjoyed playing with Aidan, who was by far the best golf partner he'd ever had.

I was amused to see my *poète maudit* getting up early and polishing his clubs, ready for a round of golf with people with whom I would have thought he had nothing in common. Aidan was in many respects an older version of the Catholic public school boys I had gone out with as a teenager in London. Without knowing it, I had reverted to type: socially confident, well mannered, entertaining, with an innate passion for cricket and rugby. But never had I known a Catholic public school boy with the passion for reading and, when it could no longer be avoided, writing, that was such an essential part of Aidan.

★

We were both working on short stories, but our approaches were so far apart that there was very little common ground.

119

Mine usually started with some autobiographical incident that had puzzled me, which I tried to make sense of while rewriting it as a story. I showed him some that I was battling to get right, and had been for some years. It was a long, drawn-out process, but I enjoyed this unpressurised work. His comment in his diary (which I read only years later) was 'What on earth was that about? Those old stories, including the gang on the yacht?' Nevertheless, he typed up a helpful page of notes, pointing out clichés and other stylistic shortcomings that could be improved on. The most useful thing he homed in on, as a natural post-modernist, was my tendency to tell the story in an all-knowing narrative voice, rather than use a neutral reporting voice and let readers make what they would of the events.

When he gave me the evolving version of 'Sodden Fields' that he had been working on since arriving in Kinsale, I was puzzled by an eight-page preamble listing things that had happened in 1927. Why 1927? Then I remembered that was the year of his birth. In reply to a request to turn it into a longer story, he had tacked an unfinished piece about 1927, culled from a notebook, on to the beginning. I didn't like its total self-obsession, and didn't think it added anything to the story that followed. If anything, it diminished it. But I was very impressed with the 'main' story, and the way it intertwined Kinsale's tragic past, the Battle of Kinsale in which the old Irish order was conquered by Queen Elizabeth I's troops, with the present-day life of characters in a run-down fishing port.

On a short visit to London in March we had gone to meet Robin Robertson at Secker & Warburg's headquarters, which was then a modest Georgian town house in Soho not far from where I used to live. Robin's office was at the top of a long, carpeted staircase, lined with uniform Secker volumes. It seemed like the perfect home for Aidan's work.

Reg had negotiated a modest two-book deal, and Robin seemed genuinely keen on Aidan's work. The hope was that he would become Aidan's long-term editor, a trusted companion, helping his work to develop over the years.

Because of my decision not to read Aidan's letters, and his own disinclination to discuss the business side of his work in any detail, I didn't realise at the time that the two books that Secker was about to publish had been casualties of the demise of Allison & Busby, the publishers of *Bornholm Night-Ferry*. Bill Swainson, a contemporary of Robin's, who had known Aidan's work since starting his publishing career some ten years earlier in John Calder's office, had begun to put together two collections, one of 'Travels and Autobiographies' and one of 'Fictions and Autobiographies', for Allison & Busby at least a year before. Together the books would amount to a relaunch of Aidan's work, a chance for the reappraisal of a writer who had been in print since 1960, but whose books, while highly praised, all too often had fallen through the cracks when it came to winning the critical attention – and sales – they deserved. Following our visit to the office, a contract was drawn up. The books were to be published in 1989, the 'Travels and Autobiographies', including *Images of Africa*, collected in *Ronda Gorge & Other Precipices* in March, and the 'Fictions and Autoboigraphies' in *Helsingør Station & Other Departures* in September. Both books were dedicated 'to Alannah'.

Derek was appalled at the smallness of the advance, something he was resigned to as a poet, but he thought Aidan deserved better – and Aidan agreed. Even though he now had Reg acting for him as agent, and had already agreed to the deal Reg had brokered, he wrote to Robin:

> *You say you want to launch 'Ronda' properly, but feel that sales*
> *will not be very considerable. This seems a very lame way to*
> *begin, akin to Calder excusing poor advances by saying my work*
> *was 'difficult', which it is not. If you value the stuff, you would*
> *be able to put a decent figure on it. You have Abacus, European*
> *market, not to mention USA to cover such extravagance, if you*
> *consider it so. You are offering beginners' fees.*[9]

Aidan was asking for £5,000 for the two books, twice as much as the terms he had just agreed with Reg. Of course, Robin did not budge, and the deal went ahead on Reg's terms. Aidan's letter ended with a warm invitation to Robin to visit Kinsale, sample the local cuisine, and see for himself the house we had recently bought. 'Need funds to sink into old house, and soon,' he explained.

*

A phone call from Robin in mid-August let us know that he was planning to visit Kinsale on Friday, 2 September for two nights, to work on the editing. His wife, Clare Reihill, was arriving on Saturday evening from Dublin – could we find them somewhere nice to stay near our place?

The visit went well. We met Robin in Cork at the station in the afternoon. He and Aidan got down to work straight away in our sitting room at the Dutch House. I cooked a meal for us in the Dutch House on the first night. Robin and Aidan worked until about nine, and again the next day from about ten.

On the first night Robin queried Aidan's use of the phrase 'The music meliorated across the water,' and would not allow it. This was queried again the next day. Aidan claimed that Beckett had used the phrase to describe the improved clarity of sound that had travelled over water, but he couldn't remember where. Without an exact citation, it would not be allowed. It was agreed that 'meliorate' was a word, it was in the OED, *v. improve*; the argument was about whether it could be used of sound over water, and in Robin's opinion it could not. When Aidan discovered that Robin was from Aberdeen, he blamed his refusal to change his position on Scots stubbornness.

Both Robin and Clare were very taken with Kinsale. We walked around Compass Hill in the sun with Robin when the editing was finished, and he loved the panoramic view of the harbour. Clare arrived as we got back to town and we drove her and Robin out to the Old Head of Kinsale, stopping for a drink at the Dock Bar on our way back. They asked about house prices. He would be very tempted to give up editing and live here and write poetry, he said. Clare said she would prefer Dublin.

We had dinner at Jim Edwards' and discovered the usual web of literary connections. I was reviewing Carlo Gébler's book about Cuba for the *Irish Times*: Clare had been talking to him the week before about a script for a film she was making. From Kinsale they were heading for Dublin, where Robin would be working with John Banville on his new novel, *The Book of Evidence*. John had a new job as a subeditor at the *Irish Times*, and the novel would do extremely well.

*

I made a solemn vow that we would be living in the Higher Street house before our quarterly rent at the Dutch House became due in early November. So I decided not to take on any work other than the usual *Irish Times* book reviewing until the move had been made. Robin had asked for more pages for both the new stories, as many pages as Aidan could write, at least twenty, and Aidan, notebook in hand, was hard at work. Most mornings he was up at 5 a.m., and spent the rest of the day in a state of high excitement. He had made so many amendments to 'Sodden Fields', his Kinsale story, that the whole thirty-four-page story needed retyping. I didn't like typing at the best of times, and still lacked a decent chair and desk. I knew that Jill had typed his work, and I wasn't going to fall into that habit. But Aidan's excitement was hard to resist, and I was officially between projects, with no urgent work to hand. Aidan would wave a batch of closely amended pages at me, saying, 'See where you can fit these in.' On one day I typed twenty pages of 'The Bird I Fancied', and the next day twenty-one. My back was aching. I made a mental note not to tell him in future when I was taking a break from my own work.

In the midst of all this, I had an urgent call from London: my father had been admitted to hospital with a suspected perforated ulcer; it was an emergency, could I come over to stay with my mother until he was home again? I could, of course, and was only too glad to be able to help. My father was home within the week, but was still very frail, and my mother too, so I stayed for a fortnight.

When I got back to Kinsale, Aidan had hardly slept, and 'The Bird I Fancied' was now a chaotic ninety-five pages long. He gave it to me, and asked if I could disentangle it. I gave it back with suggestions for some cuts, and several large chunks transposed. This time Aidan did the typing, and finally the stories were finished and sent off to Secker.

I had to make up for lost time on the house, and immediately organised a local builder to concrete the muddy back yard, and remove the decking. It was a good start. Then I heard that my cousin Tubby, a carpenter, was out of work, so I asked him to work for us for as long as it took to get the house in order. At the same time I asked the Great O'Leary to quote for the painting. He and Tubby got on famously, and the whole house was repainted, the floors sanded, and a bookcase and two desks built, in less than a week.

There was a huge sense of goodwill towards the new house: everything seemed to fall into place as if pre-ordained. We moved in on Saturday, 5 November 1988, just short of the second anniversary of our meeting on 18 November 1986. Even though we were exhausted, we played an inaugural game of Scrabble in front of a blazing fire in the wood-burning stove.

We had our house-warming party at 12.30 p.m. the next day. Nearly everyone we knew came along, or so it seemed. Tomás brought a bottle of Black Bushmills, which he then proceeded to drink – not a good idea. Desmond O'Grady came with Ellen, heavily pregnant, and two small dogs. Katherine and Joachim brought their children, who explored the garden. Stan remarked that the house move had made my hair turn grey; in fact I was experimenting – it was meant to look distinguished. The gallant Peter Murray commented, 'Stan is one of the rudest men I've ever met,' and I agreed. When the drink ran out, we went down to Jim Edwards' with the stragglers, and drank one last toast to our new home.

On Monday Aidan's diary notes that he 'picked up the first post in 2 Higher Street. Had a Radox bath, listening to a robin carolling in garden, jackdaws and crows in dispute or accord among the roof tiles and chimney pots.'

We were both surprised by the difference it made, having a house and a garden of our own, being homeowners for the first time. A whole world of domesticity suddenly took on a new interest. We spent hours wandering around hardware shops, tile shops, carpet showrooms, garden centres and paint shops, even the homeware department of Dunnes

Stores, none of which had hitherto held any attraction. We both found enormous pleasure in the house, in owning it together, cleaning it together, decorating it together, buying things for it together.

Aidan was reading the letters of Freya Stark, and found a quote that he liked: 'There is a mysterious pleasure in owning a scrap of earth far greater than any other possession. I wonder why.'

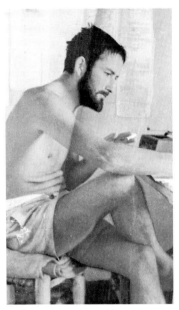

Aidan in Nerja, early 1960s.

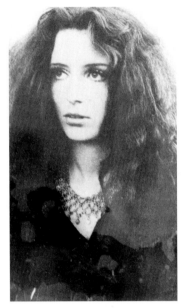

In the Desierto de los Leones, Mexico City, 1970.

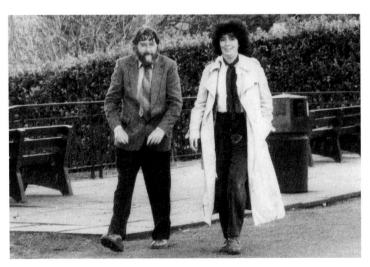

Leaving the zoo together, Dublin, 1987. Photograph courtesy of Bill Swainson.

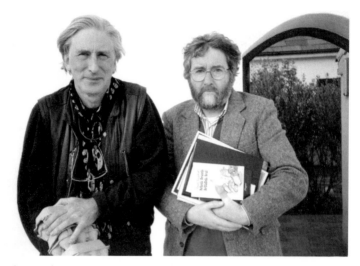

Aidan with Tomi Ungerer, Dunlough, Mizen Head, County Cork, 1988.

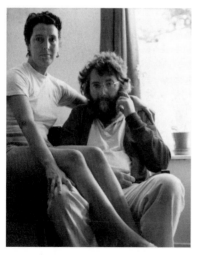

At the Dutch House, Kinsale, 1987.

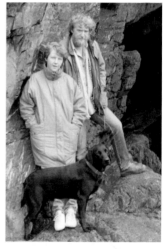

Dermot Healy, Helen and Chalkey, Nohoval Cove, County Cork, 1988.

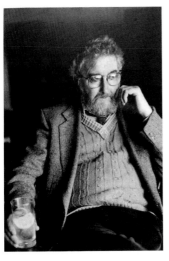

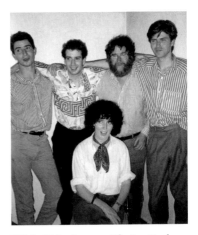

With Aidan's sons, Elwin, Carl and Julien, London, 1989.

Aidan at home with gin and tonic, Kinsale, 1990. Photograph © John Minihan.

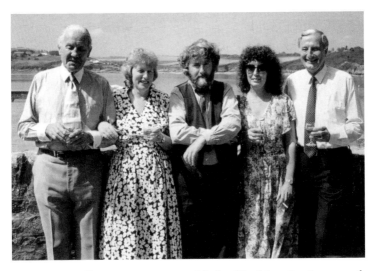

On the seawall in Summercove with the Hopkins: Pa, Jenny and Denis, 1990.

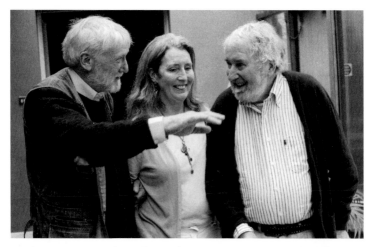

With Dermot Healy at the 'Aidan Higgins at 80' Weekend,
Celbridge, County Kildare, May 2007. Photograph © John Minihan.

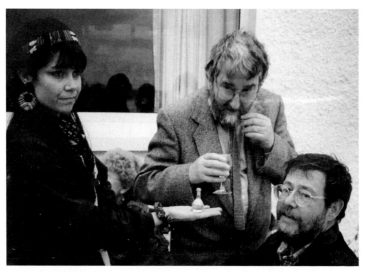

Aidan with Penelope Collins and Barry Cooke at Rosses Point
after scattering the ashes of Patrick Collins (Penelope's father) in
the Garavogue, June 1994. Some of Patrick's ashes are kept in the
little jar that Penelope holds in her hand.

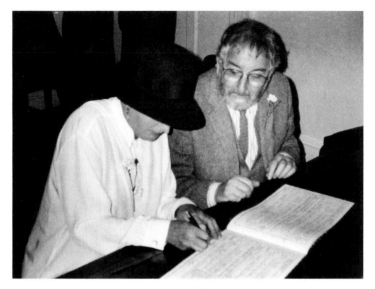

Signing the marriage register, Dublin, 20 November 1997.

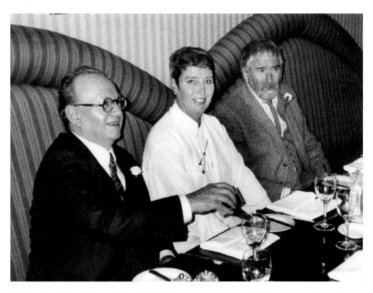

With the Best Man, Derek Mahon, at our wedding reception in
Buswell's Hotel.

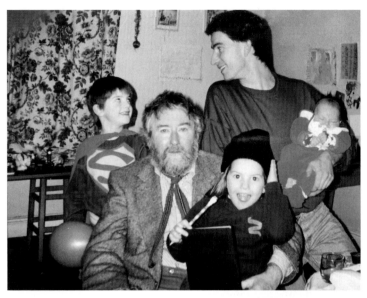

Aidan with his son, Elwin, and grandchildren, Paris, Yanika and Oscar, December 1994.

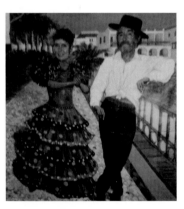

Posing as flamenco dancers, Nerja, 1999.

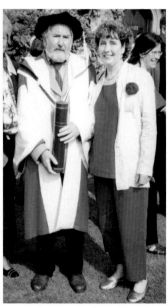

Conferred as an Honorary Doctor of Letters, University College Cork, May 2003.

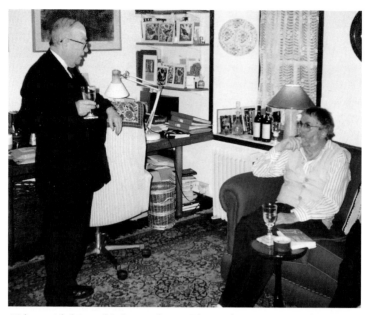

Aidan with his publisher, John Calder, at home in Kinsale, 2006.

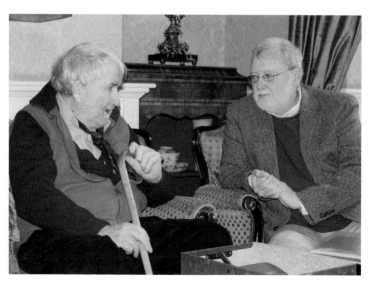

And with his publisher, John O'Brien of Dalkey Archive Press, in Buswell's Hotel, Dublin, 2010.

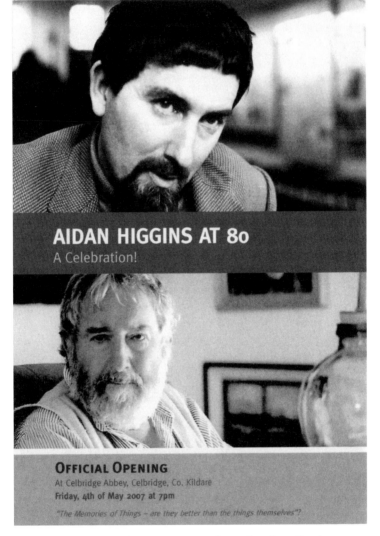

AIDAN HIGGINS AT 80
A Celebration!

OFFICIAL OPENING
At Celbridge Abbey, Celbridge, Co. Kildare
Friday, 4th of May 2007 at 7pm

"The Memories of Things – are they better than the things themselves"?

The flyer for the 'Aidan Higgins at 80' Weekend, Celbridge, County Kildare, May 2007.

PART II
A Very Long Honeymoon
1989–98

In March 1988, Vincent Dowling, Artistic Director of the Abbey Theatre, had written to Aidan about his proposed play, *Assassin*: 'I read your script without leaving it down. It is certainly the most extraordinary script it has ever been my good fortune to read! Let us meet as soon as possible.' Aidan noted in his diary a few days later that he was 'mistrustful' of Dowling's letter. Perhaps he was thinking of the anecdote in Lauren Bacall's autobiography about the Broadway producer who always heaped praise on plays that he knew were no good. Further communication from Dowling said that he would give it a 'rehearsed reading' when the Abbey's company was touring with *The Playboy of the Western World*. 'The actors like to have something to do while they are touring, it stops them from getting bored.'

Almost a year later came confirmation that the rehearsed reading would take place in Cork on Tuesday, 7 February 1989 at 2 p.m. in the Triskel Arts Centre. It was also the opening night of the Cork leg of their tour; tickets would be left for us at the box office. As my car was once again being repaired, we went up to Cork on the 10.30 bus on a drizzly day. We were early, so we indulged our current hobby: buying things for our house. We went to the brass shop and bought a brass porthole, a brass doorknob, a knocker in the shape of a lion, and a letterbox. They were all for our front door.

Aidan and I were the only guests at the Triskel, we sat with Vincent Dowling, and were formally welcomed by the actor John Olohan. The company sat around a large table and read from their scripts with terrific animation. The play was much better than we had expected, carried largely by the character of Princip (the assassin) and the actors' commitment. The two women in the cast were full of praise, especially for the language of the play, and Vincent Dowling was visibly affected. Dowling had to return to Dublin by train, and nothing was decided. The drizzle had now turned into a downpour, so a car was called for Dowling, who gave us a lift as far as the Oyster Tavern, a traditional Cork seafood restaurant. We had a leisurely pre-theatre dinner of whitebait and Muscadet. We were both pleasantly surprised by the actors' enthusiasm for the script, but also sceptical of Dowling's intention to take it any further. Aidan found him affected, and called him a calculating careerist. But, he said, he told a good story. Dowling was of course a Dubliner, a city with a celebrated tradition of anecdotalising. He had a reputation as a womaniser; maybe that was why I instinctively disliked him. He asked whether I wrote poetry, but did not seem to know that I reviewed theatre. No one had mentioned my surname, so perhaps he assumed it was Higgins. In contrast, we were both very taken with Peadar Lamb and John Olohan, down-to-earth theatre people with the courtly manners of a previous age.

It was a full house and the interval was unusually lively. The bar at Cork Opera House ran the length of the front of the building, behind the auditorium itself. As a consequence it had two entrances, one at either side, and was an excellent place to meet people. Aidan thought he spotted the poet John Montague, and immediately ducked out of one door, and scooted across the lobby to the far side of the bar. And who did he run into there, but Evelyn Montague, John's rather formidable Parisian wife, whom Aidan referred to as Madame Montague, having once addressed her as Madeleine, the name of the wife before. The two couples had been friends while Aidan was still living with Jill, and the Montagues had often stayed in the Muswell Hill flat. Evelyn introduced her eldest daughter, Oonagh, and we all shook hands. When Aidan said he thought he'd just seen John on the far side of the bar, Evelyn assured Aidan that 'the poet', as she called him in a mildly sarcastic tone, was in America. The poet was in Brooklyn; it was yet another case of mistaken identity, or a '*doppelgänger*', as Aidan called it, something that often seemed to happen to him. He and John had come to blows some years earlier in London, in the apartment at Muswell Hill, and had avoided each other ever since. Aidan admitted he had been taking some kind of speed, and had just flipped when Montague turned up yet again to have supper and stay the night without contributing a bottle, and could not resist the compulsion to punch him in the face. I thought it was a strange way for grown men to behave. I neither liked nor disliked John Montague; he had always been polite and helpful to me. When my tutoring hours at UCC were cut, he suggested that I apply for a PhD under his supervision: I would have an income, and he would leave me free to write my own work. But I knew that if I applied for a PhD on an academic topic (the only option back then) I would end up writing on that topic, and not doing my own work.

We had been invited backstage after the show. Aidan was immediately encircled by admirers, including two very pretty young ones with long curly hair. John Olohan spoke of the possibility of a small-scale production of *Assassin* for the Abbey's experimental stage, the Peacock, which seemed a more realistic option than Dowling's grandiose plans. Peadar Lamb was staying in Kinsale for the run of the play and offered us a lift home. It turned out he was staying in our nearest pub, the Folk House, and that he was actually younger than Aidan, though he looked much older. He had known Aidan's early mentors, Arland Ussher and Arthur Power, and was also a friend of the novelist Ralph Cusack. When we reached Kinsale, Aidan and Peadar went into the Folk House, on the strength of Peadar being a resident and therefore able to buy drink, to continue the conversation about old times, while I went home to bed.

*

The Kinsale Arts Week, which had been set up on a wing and a prayer the year before, had turned out to be highly successful, and the town's tourist businesses – especially the publicans – had realised its potential for attracting visitors, so there was to be another one in 1989. The committee was voluntary, though we would have a paid festival manager nearer the date. I had agreed to programme the art events as well as the readings, so there was a meeting of one sort or another for me to attend every week. Aidan resented my absence because it interfered with our Scrabble schedule, but I assured him it would not go on forever.

I knew Aidan and I did not agree on everything, but I did not yet know the limits of our disagreements. Music definitely had potential for many disagreements. It meant very little to Aidan, while it means a lot to me. But I would never expect to meet anyone who shared all my musical tastes, which range from country music to Irish traditional, flamenco and Fado, to Baroque music on original instruments, opera, Sibelius, Mahler, Borodin,

Shostakovich, and the mainstream classical repertoire, including contemporary classical, especially guitar, which I had played until quite recently. Aidan and I were from different generations, but there was some common ground: the Gypsy Kings, Bob Marley, Bach's cello suites and the classical guitar repertoire. Soon after we met, we drove two hours to Limerick and stayed the night so that I could hear the Czech guitarist Vladimir Mikulka perform. I had discovered his music at a guitar summer school in 1984. Aidan liked most of the guitar repertoire. He also liked music sung in Spanish, and would often dance along to it. He was a good dancer, restrained but rhythmic, and light on his feet.

But he loathed Bob Dylan, having been subjected to 'Sad-Eyed Lady of the Lowlands' on repeat by a friend in Nerja. Neither did he have any time for the other 'greats' that I had grown up with in the 1960s and 1970s – Buddy Holly, Roy Orbison, the Beatles, the Rolling Stones, Muddy Waters, Leadbelly, Janice Joplin, Leonard Cohen, Ry Cooder and so on – none of them meant anything to him. We were briefly friends with Ray Davies of The Kinks, who lived in Kinsale for a while in the 1990s. Aidan could name several of his songs, greatly to my surprise. 'Waterloo Sunset', 'Sunny Afternoon', 'Dedicated Follower of Fashion'. It turned out that he had been introduced to The Kinks by his sons. Ray Davies and his brother Dave were among the few famous people to have come out of Muswell Hill. Aidan never called him Ray, but always referred to him in the singular as 'the Kink'.

★

Grafton had employed a publicist to coordinate the launch of the St Patrick book, which was scheduled for 9 March.

My two previous books had been published in London, with the minimum of ceremony – lunch with the publisher, dinner with my agent, and then the long wait for reviews. The day after our night at the theatre, my publicist rang to say that Peter Harbison, Professor of Archaeology at Trinity College Dublin, had read the page proofs, and rang to let her know how much he liked the book. The omens were good. She wanted me to provide a guest list for the launch at Waterstone's in Cork, still a novelty, since it had opened only the year before. I would have preferred the Collins Bookshop, whose owner Con was always good to us, but Waterstone's was bigger, so Waterstone's it had to be.

My parents came over from London especially, and a large crowd of friends and relations from Kinsale, Cork and Dublin assembled in Waterstones, along with several men in suits from Grafton, and the publicist. My mother had kindly taken me shopping for 'an outfit', but nothing appealed. Instead, I wore a long black cotton dress by Vivienne Westwood that my niece Gabriela had bought some years before, with my mother's Kinsale cloak (lined with bright-green silk), and her Tara brooch on the front of the dress. Aidan was intermittently at my side, leaving me plenty of space to circulate. One of my friends told me Aidan was obviously 'over the moon'. 'You must be very proud of your daughter,' someone said to my parents. 'We are,' they said, beaming.

When we saw them off at Cork airport my mother, who knew she did not have much longer to live, said to Aidan, 'In case I don't see you again, thank you for looking after Alannah.' As she spoke, he said the shadow of a departing jet crossed her face. I suppose your youngest child will always need looking after, even if she will be forty next birthday. My parents had decided to leave my father's car, a Peugeot 504, in Ireland. When they were not here, the large, comfortable and relatively new car was ours.

The reviews were good: the book was the first study to explain the origins of the iconography of St Patrick – an old man in bishop's robes for the Catholics, and a young Roman soldier in sandals for the Protestants. Kevin Myers in the *Irish Times*'s 'Irishman's Diary' asked, 'Is this the most important book of 1989?' to which Stan, true to form, commented sourly 'It's only March.' Aidan, who had two books coming out later that year, *Ronda Gorge & Other Precipices* in March and *Helsingør Station & Other Departures* in September, said nothing. One of the locals in the Bulman, a Cork businessman, heard me on the radio, and declared that I had a very photogenic voice, which delighted Aidan.

Next Saturday it was Aidan's turn: a review of the travel writing, *Ronda Gorge & Other Precipices*, by William Trevor was published in the *Irish Times*. It concluded: 'Good writing is an act of transformation, the ordinary made fascinating, magic without tricks. That act is repeatedly performed in *Ronda*. The skill and precision that accompany it, the subtlety of its impressionistic communication, are consistently a pleasure.' Aidan thought the review lacked excitement. He said, 'I've never felt less about a book coming out.'

The review was accompanied by an advertisement for readings with Aidan, John Banville and the poet Matthew Sweeney in Dublin and then Belfast. Reading tours were still quite a novelty, and this one, organised by Robin Robertson, and featuring three Secker authors, was considered highly unusual.

The next Tuesday we set off for Dublin in the Peugeot. Because Belfast was so far from Kinsale, we had decided that, rather than travel by train, we would take the car and extend the trip after the reading to visit friends, which I would then write up as a travel piece. I arranged complimentary hotels in Bushmills and Derry, but left the last night open. The reading at Trinity in the Jonathan Swift Theatre in the Arts Building attracted a large crowd. Aidan referred to Robin as the ringmaster of the Secker circus, with his well-prepared introductions. Aidan read first, then Matthew Sweeney, who seemed very young and very nervous. John Banville read very well, as always, but for rather longer than the twenty minutes allotted. I sat next to his wife Janet, who laughed at the appropriate times, and applauded enthusiastically. I took note of this, as proper wifely behaviour.

The reception afterwards in the Douglas Hyde Gallery, a basement space in the Arts Building, was a bit eerie; the space was a gallery for contemporary art, and not really suitable; it was like being in an empty warehouse. Aidan was immediately surrounded by admirers, so I left him and chatted with Colman and Sylvia, who had made a rare trip to Dublin for the occasion. Sylvia was wearing an extraordinary red velvet cocktail hat with a full-face net, and matching 1940s-style dress. She told me she had steamed the hat specially for the occasion, but was not sure if it was the right thing: she had no idea what one wore to a reading, never having been to one before. I noticed Aidan carefully avoiding Francis Stuart (whose politics and writing he loathed) and Paul Durcan, who were chatting with young Sweeney, as he called Matthew.

We ended up in O'Neills pub, a noisy student joint, with a small crowd of friends, including Aidan's former editor, Bill Swainson, from London, and Bernard and Elizabeth Share. We continued on to Buswells Hotel, where Robin was staying, but were refused admission on the grounds that it was now after hours, and we were not hotel guests.

I was, as often, amazed at Aidan's stamina: we had started out in Kinsale early that morning, driven for nearly four hours, had drinks before the reading, he'd given the reading, then visited two more bars, and was still keen to go on. But Dublin licensing laws prevailed, and we got a taxi to our guest house near Lansdowne Road.

The next day was a rest day for the writers, before the Belfast reading on the Thursday. The only obligation was to drop in at Buswells, and sign some fifty copies of *32 Counties*, a book of photographs of Ireland by Donovan Wylie that Secker was publishing. I arranged to meet Aidan at noon in Davy Byrne's. The guitarist Vladimir Mikulka was playing that night at the Royal Hospital Kilmainham, and I wanted to buy tickets, and also to tour the bookshops. *The Living Legend of St Patrick* was in most windows, and beside the tills. In Fred Hanna's, Aidan's book and mine were together at the till, which was very nice to see. *The Book of Evidence* by John Banville, by far the most commercial of the three Secker titles, dominated their displays.

Aidan had run into Bill Swainson on Stephen's Green, and the pair of them turned up at Davy Byrne's. The plan was to visit Dublin Zoo, and Aidan invited Bill along, 'If I'm not intruding?' he said.

I had discovered that the zoo and the Botanical Gardens at Glasnevin were Aidan's preferred way of passing the time if he had to spend a day in Dublin, because it kept him out of the pubs. As it turned out, this was the last time we went to the zoo, where we stayed for two hours, looking at the animals in their cages. Many of them were now commercially sponsored, to Aidan's horror. The beautiful snow leopard, for example, all the way from Tibet, was sponsored by Kool for Katz hairdressers. Others were just plain sad – the lone African elephant, the neurotic polar bears walking round and round in circles in their compound designed by Colman's mentor, Lubetkin. Bill took a photograph of Aidan and me leaving the zoo, which became a favourite of ours, one of very few ever taken of us as a couple.

We left for Belfast the next morning with Theo Dorgan, whom we had met by chance the evening before, in the back seat. He was pleasant company, better than a car radio, chatting away about mutual acquaintances. He also gave me invaluable directions for getting out of Dublin. We all hated the tension of the border crossing; these were very tense times. It was while we were being eyed by surly customs officers guarded by heavily armed, very young soldiers that I remembered we were travelling in a UK-registered car, and I only had an Irish driving licence with my Kinsale address. Fortunately, we were waved through, and no questions asked.

Belfast was a bit flat after Dublin. There was a wine reception near Queen's University in an untidy bookshop, scheduled to start two hours before the reading. The wine reception usually happened after a reading, not before. There was speculation that this was a Northern ruse to get the southern writers drunk before the event, and they all vowed to foil the plan by being unusually abstemious. About thirty people gathered for the reading in a small, cold, steeply raked lecture hall, in an otherwise empty building. Edna Longley welcomed the visitors on behalf of Queen's English Society, while Robin introduced the writers. Edna's husband, the poet Michael Longley, whom we had met in Kinsale with Derek, was very attentive. Banville seemed to read better every time I heard him, while Matthew seemed just as nervous. 'Give them Hell, young Sweeney,' Aidan hissed in his ear as he went up to read. There seemed to be nowhere to go afterwards but back to our hotel, with a dozen or so friends.

On Friday morning we parted company with the Secker people and set off on our own tour of Northern Ireland. We were going to lunch with an architect friend of mine in Islandmagee, then drive up through the Glens of Antrim to stay at the Bushmills Inn. On Saturday, God knows why, we spent the night in an extremely tense Derry city. Aidan never left the hotel. I did a circuit of the town centre, and failed to find a single bookshop. We were kept awake much of the night by loud wedding guests gallivanting in the corridor. Sometimes I become very English: I wanted to open the door and tell them to be quiet, people were trying to sleep. But Aidan absolutely forbade any such intervention, because we were in the North. Consider it a war zone, he said. He blocked my way to the door, looking frightened, so I backed down.

Aidan woke up in a bad temper. I reckoned he was exhausted. We ordered a continental breakfast in the room, in order to make a quick getaway. We left for Omagh, where we were going to lunch with Aidan's friend the artist Philomena Rafferty, who had moved back home after retiring from the civil service in London. He had been introduced to her by Gerard Dillon when he first went to London, as someone who would help him find his way around, and she had been a good friend to him and to Jill. Every Christmas she sent Aidan a lino cut of a wading bird, and he had kept them all; we had them framed and they hung on our staircase.

We forgot to change money before leaving the hotel, and set out into the Northern Ireland Sunday morning, when only hotels were open, with only 54 pence in cash. We saw many churchgoers, but no hotels, where we could change our Irish punts for sterling, until we reached Omagh. Aidan left me sipping milky coffee in a stuffy hotel lounge, and came back with an *Observer* and a *Sunday Tribune*. There were no reviews of *Ronda*. He had encountered a heavily armed foot patrol, which had shaken him badly.

Philomena was living with her older sister, Agnes, a far more conventional woman, recently retired after a life working in Toronto. They shared a modern bungalow; that is to say, Agnes had the bungalow, while Phil had converted the double garage into her quarters, a book-filled space lined with paintings by Gerard Dillon and herself. She and Colman had studied watercolour painting with Dillon in Connemara. She had installed a shower, a kitchenette, and a small TV, and said she had all that she needed, and could go for days without seeing Agnes. Aidan thought the arrangement very unfair.

Aidan was especially taken with her painting of clothes drying on a washing line, but Philomena said it wasn't for sale. We ate lunch in her sister's dining room, with family silver, crystal glasses and crocheted antimacassars on the chintz armchairs. Philomena opened a second bottle of wine as we ate the delicious roast lamb she had cooked. Agnes assured Aidan that the heavily armed young soldiers in the foot patrols were doing a great job, and were far more impartial than the RUC: 'They are very welcome here. Without them we'd be in a blood bath; it'd be all-out civil war.'

When we left at 4.30 p.m., after coffee and cake, we were offered sandwiches for the road, just as my mother would have done.

We were heading south, aiming to cross the border into Cavan. Aidan was sad at seeing Philomena in such uncongenial circumstances. He thought she would have been better off to have stayed in London, where she had friends and a lively cultural life. Omagh, he said, was worse than the end of the world, and Agnes was a bully and a bore. Beyond Belcoo, absorbed in conversation, we suddenly realised we had driven into a roadblock, jeeps parked in chevrons across the road, a gut-wrenching moment, but we were simply waved through. We were both glad to cross the border, relaxing again at the mucky road verges, the potholes and the safety of the known.

It was getting late, and I was tired of driving. The plan had been to push on to Galway city, but in Claremorris we found a bar with a restaurant and 'rooms', decorated with sumptuous red velvet upholstery, and many mirrors in what Aidan called 'brothel-style'.

'The pub has always been here, but the hotel is new,' the owner explained to us. We lounged back on the heap of cushions, and flicked through the British channels on our television, a rare novelty, as we didn't have one at home. We were both tired, and we slept early.

There was a folk club and disco behind the bar that we hadn't been told about: at 3 a.m. we were woken by a roar of 'The Fields of Athenry', seemingly sung by a massed male-voice choir. I looked out of the window and saw the street alive with cheerful lads, one standing on top of a red car, leading the singing. Contrary to what we read in the newspapers, the youth of Mayo had not emigrated; they were all at the disco in Claremorris, having harmless fun. It was good to be home.

★

When *Helsingør Station & Other Departures* came out in September, there were two reviews that Aidan became

obsessed about: Eileen Battersby's in the *Irish Times* and
Aisling Maguire's in the *Sunday Tribune*. Both were short,
unenthusiastic pieces. Both objected to the story title 'The
Bird I Fancied' and did not like his elliptical way of writing. He
lumped these two reviewers together as 'the Dublin feminists',
and complained for many years that 'the Dublin feminists'
had ganged up on him. He wrote to Eileen about her review,
singling out her abbreviation of the book's title in the review's
heading to 'Helsingør Station', as an insult. It was of course
not her responsibility, which I pointed out, but he was not
interested. To his mind it was an insult, and that was that.

Her lukewarm reception of the book was immediately
apparent: 'this more than curious collection of bits and
pieces, some of which give the impression of having been
salvaged from the cutting-room floor'. She gives faint
praise to 'Killachter Meadow' and '*Lebensraum*'. She had
obviously read no further than the opening section of
'Sodden Fields', since she referred to the story as 'a not
entirely successful celebration of and/or requiem for the
year of his birth, 1927'. 'The Bird I Fancied' is referred to as
'unfortunately titled' (apparently the affectionate cockney
use of 'bird' had failed to travel), and, she concluded, 'leaves
the reader bludgeoned by the rampant ego of the narrator's
self-obsession'. She did, however, have high praise for the
story 'Frère Jacques, Bruder Jacques', which she judged to
be 'tightly focused, uncluttered by a harsh slickness which
appears to be threatening his style'. Many writers have had
worse reviews than that, but for whatever reason Aidan
took it very badly.

I was advised early on by my neighbour Robert Nye,
author of *Falstaff* (among other fine historical novels), and a
fellow Hamish Hamilton author, to count the column inches
when reading reviews, and pay no attention at all to what they

said, be it good or bad. But Aidan didn't think like this, and nothing I could say would reconcile him to what he saw as a major slight. He never got over those two reviews. I don't think his resentment had anything to do with the fact that both Derek and I knew Eileen, and enjoyed her company. Some fourteen years after the event, Aidan specifically recalled the review in a letter to the *Irish Times*, bemoaning the harsh treatment by critics of his work, referring to Eileen, who was by then the *Irish Times*' 'Literary Correspondent', as 'your acid resident American critic'. Eileen told me that she had received acrimonious letters from Aidan at intervals for years after.

This was also the start of a long-running correspondence between Aidan and the *London Review of Books*. I don't have a copy of the first letter he wrote to them, complaining about the lack of reviews, nor of Mary Kay Wilmers' reply. On 27 November 1989, he transcribes in his diary, without comment, a reply from Mary Kay Wilmers to another letter of his:

> *Dear Mr Higgins,*
> *What I said was that I was appalled that you should think we had a conspiracy against you, which is different. I am sorry your books were not reviewed, but we can't I'm afraid, go back to them now.*
> *Yours sincerely*
> *Mary Kay Wilmers*

He continued to complain to Mary Kay about the *LRB*'s failure to review his books for the rest of his working life. It is clear from Mary Kay's consistently polite replies that it was a genuine accident. His books were sent out for review by the literary editor, in mixed batches, and it was up to the reviewer to choose which ones to write about. On another occasion a major reassessment was commissioned but never written. He felt this neglect acutely, and saw it as a deliberate slight, no matter what anybody said. I think it was just unfortunate, just one of those things. *The Times Literary Supplement*, however, which is a weekly publication with a different remit, faithfully commissioned and ran a review of every single book by Aidan, as it was published, as well as occasional longer overviews.

A cutting pasted in the same page of Aidan's 1989 diary as the letter from Mary Kay Wilmers reads: 'The £50,000 GPA Book Award has been won by the *Irish Times'* literary editor, John Banville, for *The Book of Evidence*. The announcement was made in Dublin last night by the sole adjudicator, the novelist Graham Greene...'

The next day Aidan sent a postcard to John Banville with congratulations on the 'superloot'. The new GPA Book Award of £50,000 was a huge sum of money in 1989, at a time when the Booker Prize was worth only £21,000. *The Book of Evidence* went on to be shortlisted for the Booker Prize, further adding to its sales. In 2005 Banville finally won the Booker Prize for his thirteenth novel, *The Sea*. Once again, Aidan sent a congratulatory postcard. The acolyte, who generously acknowledged his debt to Aidan, had overtaken the master. 'Without *Langrishe, Go Down*, there would have been no *Birchwood*', he said to me once.

★

I don't know what went wrong with *Ronda Gorge & Other Precipices* (Travels & Autobiographies, 1958–89), nor its companion volume, *Helsingør Station & Other Departures* (Fictions & Autobiographies, 1958–89). They were beautifully produced books, with intricately designed dust jackets showing illustrations by Robin Cracknell, featuring scraps of Aidan's handwriting and a collage of period photos, compasses and postcards. But they didn't sell, and weren't published individually in paperback, though a selection of the pieces from each was included in an omnibus paperback of Aidan's 'short fiction' called *Flotsam and Jetsam* in 1996. Already in that collection it was becoming apparent that Aidan's preference is tending towards autobiography rather than ficiton. Nor did any foreign rights sell, unlike *Felo de Se, Langrishe, Go Down* and some of the other books published by John Calder. It seemed that the reading public was not prepared to spend money on collections of short pieces by a writer few had heard of, and if they had heard of him, it was that he was 'difficult'. Both books were remaindered two years later, as is the custom. Aidan noted the date sourly in his diary. No matter how many times people explained to him that being remaindered was common practice, he took it as a personal insult, and brooded over it for years.

Robin tried several times over the next few years to encourage Aidan to write more stories, but it was not to be. When Aidan suggested in January 1990 that his *Collected Criticism* could be his next book, Robin wrote in reply:

> *It would be a grave error for you to publish another retrospective volume at this stage. Your Collected Criticism might sell 300 copies. You must use the two Secker books as a springboard for new work, and a collection of three long pieces of fiction would certainly prompt an advance from me. To go backwards now would be an appalling mistake and a very clear signal of a career ended. The work you did on 'Sodden Fields' and 'The Bird I Fancied' shows a talent undimmed* [underlined by Aidan]. *I cannot understand why you want to stop now.*

Those two stories, completed soon after his arrival in Kinsale, are in fact the last two stories Aidan ever wrote. He was sixty. From then on, apart from the comic novel *Lions of the Grunewald* (1993), it would all be autobiography.

Writing as good as his does not come easily. When he was working on something, he put in long days at the desk in total silence. The notebooks were read and marked up, and suitable sections typed up on a manual typewriter, added to whatever he was writing, then reread closely over a couple of days, annotated, sometimes literally cut up, and paragraphs pasted into new places, then the whole freshly typed again. Everything fed into what he was working on, his walking, the daytime pub sessions, his reading, both specific and casual, newspaper headlines for example, 'Oxx has the Form', or a song called 'The Crossbarry Queer', or simply what he saw out of the window – 'Jackdaws nestled in the limes of Friary hill'. One of his favourite sayings was 'Nothing is ever wasted': as a writer everything can be recycled, slotted in, used somehow, but he took this practice to new extremes. People's life stories were listened to with unusual attention and found their place: the Great O'Leary in an Israeli Kibbutz, Mattie Maunsell who lost a lion in Inchicore, the Trapper Joe Revatta, who once caught a fleeing hare in his arms. And somehow all the bits and pieces would cohere and add up to more than the sum of their parts, often puzzling, even challenging as narrative, with a total disregard for chronology, but somehow approximating lived experience. It was a highly intuitive process and resulted in a strange kind of literary alchemy. John Banville has a neat summary of his writing style: 'Higgins' abiding characteristics as an artist are of a High Modernist order: obsessive subjectivity, a broad range of allusive references, insistence on formal freedom, a plethora of polyglottal quotations, aristocratic disdain of the audience.'[1]

Aidan's excitement at discovering a new way of writing with 'Sodden Fields' is expressed in an interview he gave in

May 1989 to an Austrian student, Ursula Mayrhuber, of the University of Vienna:

> I was asked to produce twenty pages in a week and I said, no, I couldn't do that. So I was given a fortnight, but not a day more. And I began working over in Kinsale in a way I have never worked before since I began writing. The Hidden Prompter was beginning to speak to me. I got a voice which was not male or female or living or dead. It said into my ear one morning, 'Tiny Bodini has no peace because of the magnitude of his task.' I was getting up at five in the morning and working till about two the next morning. And instead of 20 pages, I gave him 160 pages. I think this is possibly the most interesting work I have done yet. It's the first time I've been able to live in a place and write about it without hiding and camouflaging, because I think I am happy in a certain way I was not happy before, here in Kinsale.[2]

The story of Tiny Bodini crops up several times in the specially written papers that Aidan read at various festivals over the next ten years, and is told again in the third volume of memoirs, *The Whole Hog*, where the term 'the Hidden Prompter' is attributed to Saul Bellow, who coined it. (The estimate of 160 pages instead of twenty is an exaggeration. It may have felt like 160, but it was about 30.) I prefer the less intricately worked, more conversational version recorded by Mayrhuber to the more literary one Aidan wrote ten years later for *The Whole Hog*.

★

Shortly after Ursula's visit we had a fright one morning when Aidan woke up and could hardly stand for dizziness. I escorted him down to the doctor's surgery, a short walk from our house, where it was discovered that his blood pressure was dangerously high. Within hours he was an in-patient in Cork Regional Hospital under Dr Peter Kearney, younger brother of the philosopher Richard Kearney.

Aidan had been overdoing the physical work in his newly acquired garden, heaving huge rocks around, and it had taken a toll. After an angiogram it was discovered that he did not need a by-pass, but he was put on beta-blockers. It was the first time he had been in a hospital since his stay in Clonskeagh Fever Hospital in his early twenties, suffering from scarlet fever and malnutrition. He was sixty-two years old.

In November 1989, I went to see my parents in London. My mother was still in the care of my ever-patient father, who was obviously feeling the strain. She had had another series of small strokes, which had led to disphasia, the inability to find the right words, as well as the tendency to lose her bearings. But she seemed physically much better, and in very good humour, just gently going ga-ga.

At the end of my ten-day visit, my father drove the three of us to the tube station, and parked on a double yellow line. He helped to get my bag out of the boot, and kissed me goodbye.

As he got back into the car, my mother was trying to open her door to get out and say goodbye. We were causing an obstruction, and people were starting to hoot. I pushed the door closed, and leant in the window:

'Don't bother to get out. We can say goodbye from here.'

Tears were streaming down her face.

'I'll be back in January,' I said. 'I'm not going far. You can always phone me. I'll see you soon.' I air-kissed her through the window.

'I won't be here then. This is the last time I'll ever see you.'

'Now don't be silly. None of that nonsense. Cheer up. Have a good Christmas. I'll see you in January. Big kiss.'

★

Christmas 1989
Alannah to Aidan:
The Mosquito Coast by Paul Theroux
The Natural History of Selborne by Gilbert White

Aidan to Alannah:
The Secret Agent by Joseph Conrad
Giacomo Joyce by James Joyce
The Complete Stories of Elizabeth Bowen
The Fruit, Herbs and Vegetables of Italy by Giacomo Castelvetro

★

The first phone call came on Tuesday morning, 26 December, from my brother. My mother had had a stroke that morning, while my father was out, taking my sister Pixie to the tube station. She was paralysed down one side, her speech badly affected, but still seemed lucid. I rang her sister Sheila to let her know. I heard on the news that Samuel Beckett, the Irish writer, aged eighty-two, had died in a hospital in Paris. We listened to the midnight news, but got no more detail than that.

The second phone call came at 2.30 a.m. that night, 27 December. It was Pa to say that my mother's heart had stopped beating in her sleep. He had gone home at the suggestion of the medical team at midnight, leaving her alone. My brother Denis was on his way up from Purley. Pa couldn't decide whether to go to the hospital 'to see her one more time' or not. I suggested he stay put until Denis arrived.

I went back to bed, and as I told the news to Aidan I was surprised by tears, and a heavy weight of sadness. 'She was an innocent,' Aidan said, hugging me. 'A lovely innocent.' I was certain she was at peace, no more pain, and no more anxiety; the latter had been her real torment. 'You have to make big adjustments for a death,' said Aidan. 'Make space, accept you have a gap in the place of a mother.'

Aidan made the following notes in his diary:

Doctor at 2am to say Angela died peacefully in her sleep, aged 78, after small stroke. Lil passed away in Dun Laoghaire how many years ago? May, '66 was it, year LGD came out, 23 years ago. I was in Calder's office and Beckett was shown *Irish Times* (Bernard Share) review, pushing up glasses to read. That was the time he came with friends to dinner at Adamczewski's place. McGahern left before Beckett arrived. Philomena was there, and she and Fiona wanted to speak to Beckett. He sat with us, ruffled his feathers, like an eagle, he was 61, some of his best work still ahead. Calder had to get his feet into small car after much whiskey. 'There's more to publishing than just bringing out books,' Calder's comment.

…

'Do you believe in an afterlife?
　　Mine was always that.'*

'You might say I had a happy childhood although I had little talent for happiness. My parents did everything that could be done to make a child happy, but I was often lonely.'³

If anybody was going to commit suicide, you'd think it would be Beckett, yet he hung on to the end.

'Such and more such the hubbub in his mind so-called till nothing left from deep within but only ever fainter, oh to end. No matter how no matter where. Time and grief, and self so-called. Oh all to end.'⁴

From end of *Stirrings Still*, Beckett's last words written in English. To end on 'end'.

*

After my mother's death in 1989, my father decided to sell the flat in London, and live in the house in Summercove. His eyesight was fading, and without my mother as a lookout, he could no longer drive. It seemed a good solution, and we were both glad to have him living nearby. He soon fell into a comfortable routine that revolved around Sunday lunch with me or my aunt, and a regular evening visit to

---

* Aidan made these notes (including quotes from Beckett's works shown here in italics) from memory at the time of Samuel Beckett's death. Beckett actually wrote, in *Endgame* 'Do you believe in the life to come'.

the Bulman. Ashley Good and my father took to having an evening drink together in the Bulman every day at 5.15 p.m. You could set your clock by them. They sat up at the counter, as near to the middle of the bar as possible, and each bought alternate rounds: two pints of Guinness and one short, Paddy whiskey and water. Seldom more, never less.

Joanna Good had been very upset when my mother died. She cried when she came to offer me condolences, which set me off, and for the one and only time, we embraced. Then she flinched away and said, 'I never do that'.

One autumn morning I was on my own in the house in Summercove when Joanna came over, carrying a large orange life-saving buoy, salvaged from a wreck, that was used as an ornament in their front porch. Her face was red and she was highly agitated. She asked me to take care of this life-buoy, to keep it from Ashley, and not to let her son James anywhere near it. She was not making any sense, was verging on hysteria, and I was afraid of what she might do if she went back home alone. Even though I was frightened at her obviously irrational state, I kept her talking, and walked with her across the front of the pub to her house. This attracted the attention of Willie, the ever-vigilant owner of the Bulman, who could see something was wrong. I ran up to him and told him quietly to phone Ashley at work and tell him to come home.

Joanna was taken away by the men in white coats, and never came home again. She went into residential care at a place a few miles outside town called Ballintobber Lodge. She never regained her wits. Ashley visited her every afternoon for an hour. I often wondered how he managed, what on earth they talked about, whether he attempted to amuse her, whether he told her of his daily routine, or just sat and held her hand? I thought it must be one of the most difficult things in the world to do, to keep company with someone who was not aware of who you were, or why you were there. I thought that to do that for a whole hour every day was verging on saintly. But I never spoke to Ashley about it. I was afraid he would find such questions intrusive, being from an older generation, and very reserved. Mercifully, after six months, Joanna died.

My St Patrick book had gone into paperback. It had also been published in hardback in the US, but had not sold particularly well. Reg was in discussion with various publishers about other biographies, including Daphne du Maurier's, which I would have enjoyed, but that went to the more experienced Margaret Forster.

So I decided to do something different, using another set of skills from my *Time Out* days, and write a proper guidebook to County Cork, for both locals and the increasing number of visitors. After five years of working in the strict format of the American guidebook company, Fodor's, I was keen to do some real writing, and also make use of my knowledge of Cork history. Con Collins, our bookseller friend, was keen to take the guide on for his fledgling list of publications, and I was happy to do it. I would enjoy having a local publisher, even if it meant being paid less money. There was a lot of travelling involved, mainly day trips, and I often took my father along with me, as he liked travelling as much as I did.

We offered to take my father with us on our first trip together to Nerja. It was a good idea. All three of us enjoyed it, and it made it less tense than it might have been with just the two of us, as Aidan revisited the scenes of his intense infatuation with Harriet Deck (Charlotte in *Balcony of Europe*). In fact, he was very sensitive about my feelings, and never mentioned her, though he did note in his diary (which I read much later) that he was surprised by how little feeling he had for her. They had met briefly in California on his way back from Texas in 1984.

I was interested to meet Aidan's old friends, Donal and Paulette O'Farrell, whom he had known in Dublin, and then in London, where they had a flat in Hampstead. He had a photograph of them on the cover of one of his notebooks. Paulette, a small, sun-tanned French woman with long grey hair, is apparently laughing uncontrollably while leaning on a mantelpiece. She managed to look both quite distinguished and wild. Donal, a dark-haired man with a magnificent hooked nose, stood soberly by. Aidan said they were among his oldest friends. They had married when they were very young, and Paulette had scandalised Dublin by wearing one of the first bikinis to be seen on Dollymount Strand. Now that Donal had retired as a subeditor at *The Times*, they had left Hampstead, and lived between Paris, St Amour and Nerja.

Paulette found us an apartment to rent in their building, a large one above Burriana beach with a communal swimming pool. I remember the exhilaration of the afternoon flight into Spain, snow-toppped mountains giving way to ground that looked hot and parched under the early summer sun. It was a welcome novelty to be in a dry country. Paulette showed us to our apartment, then took us over to to say hallo to Donal. The evening went well, but I sensed a certain tension between Donal and Paulette. The next day she apologised to us for having drunk too much. Aidan protested that there was nothing to apologise for, but she insisted: Donal had told her she had drunk too much and made a show of herself. Unlike Donal, she did not have another drink for the duration of our stay. I did not like this evidence of control, nor did I like Paulette boasting that Donal spoke perfect Parisian French, while her own English was heavily accented to the point of comical after over forty years of marriage, because Donal liked it that way. She apparently had trouble remembering my name, so having learnt I was a writer, she called me George Sand instead. I enjoyed that.

It was sad to see my father reading Muriel Spark in the sun, holding the book at a strange angle to maximise his peripheral vision. Aidan, who had refused to bring anything to read, picked up my copy of *The Moons of Jupiter*, and spent the rest of the holiday telling me how good Alice Munro was. I had been telling him this for some time, but only now by actually reading her did he admit that I was right. Similarly, his son Elwin, a great music lover, often complained of how difficult it was to introduce anything new to Aidan, but how nice it was, once you had conquered his resistance, to see him enjoying it – Bob Marley, for example, or the Gypsy Kings.

My father was not with us for long in Kinsale. He was diagnosed with cancer, but died at home from pneumonia quite suddenly on Easter Sunday, 1993. Our friend and GP, David Nagle, assured us that succumbing to pneumonia was preferable to letting the cancer run its course. My brother Denis and I, and my neighbour Maisie, who had been employed as his nurse, sat with him to the end in the early hours of the morning. When the undertakers came to remove his remains at dusk the next day, the whole village was shocked at the suddenness of his departure.

Less than a week after my father's death and his two funerals, one in Kinsale, one in London, I had to go on the road again to do a guidebook recce for Fodor's, which was my main source of income at that time. It was a cold, wet April, and as I drove around a new ring road in Athlone in the half-light, I cursed the Irish midlands and people who expected me to go back to work before I had finished grieving. One of the shiny new road signs had been covered in graffiti which read 'Athlone – Arsehole of the Universe!', making me smile for the first time in days.

The day after I delivered my task to Fodor's, Aidan and I took off for Menorca. I'd booked us a fortnight in a holiday village that I saw advertised in the *Observer*. It was a long shot, and involved flying via Dublin and Majorca, but it turned out to be exactly what we wanted: a quiet, low-rise holiday village, built around a tennis court and a swimming pool. It was only a short walk across a nature reserve full of loudly croaking frogs to a wild sandy beach several kilometres long. Neither of us had ever been on this kind of holiday before, but we soon got the hang of it. We had the Scrabble board with us, and I had brought fourteen books, one for each day of the holiday.

As usual, Aidan had not bothered to bring anything to read, just a notebook. But he soon discovered my copy of *HMS Surprise* by Patrick O'Brian. He liked it so much that he read it twice. Over the years he read all twenty-three novels in the Aubrey-Maturin series, twice. In similar vein, we liked the holiday so much that we went back again, for the same two weeks, to exactly the same villa, the following year.

★

For a few years, while the poet Seán Dunne was features editor of the *Irish Examiner*, I had a regular weekly column in which I interviewed people about how they spent their weekends, and then edited out my questions so that the piece was in their own voice. The people who were most interesting were obsessives; sometimes they were well known, sometimes not. Occasionally I used the column as an excuse to meet someone I wanted to know, or know better, and this was how I became friends with Yvonne Ungerer, the wife of the Alsace-born graphic artist Tomi Ungerer.

Tomi and Yvonne lived on the most southerly farm in Ireland: Dunlough, at the tip of the Mizen Peninsula. Their land included a famous landmark known as the Three Castles, a picturesque group of ruined stone castle keeps built around a lake, above the jagged rocks of the Mizen, accessible only on foot. Yvonne had been a commercial sheep farmer with a flock of more than 350 ewes, but had a much smaller herd by the time we met. Aidan called her 'the shepherdess', but she was also a highly cultured, serious woman, a dark-haired beauty with a distinctive style, wearing hand-made textiles and ethnic jewellery. Now that she had less outdoor work, she played the piano with serious application, and spent an increasing amount of time in Nepal, chanting. She had her own circle of friends, and was happy to spend time alone on the farm, while Tomi was in his birthplace, Strasbourg, furthering his career.

Tomi and Yvonne had met in New York. She was a young model who had grown up on a small farm in Connecticut, and he a successful graphic artist, considerably older. As he never tired of telling his teenage children, he had arrived in New York with sixty dollars in his pocket and nothing but his talent and the will to succeed. Both Tomi and Yvonne were soon disillusioned with city life and the commercial world, and moved to a smallholding in Nova Scotia. Tomi retained close links with Strasbourg, and in 1975 the harsh climate, and his desire to live in Europe again, led them to Ireland, where they bought Dunlough. Yvonne, who had Irish grandparents, always said there was something inevitable about their move to such an extraordinary and beautiful place. Their three children were born and reared in Ireland, and they were all very much part of the local community. At the time of our first visit there was a blackboard in the kitchen with words written in English, French and German, part of Tomi's determination that his children should grow up with the three languages that he spoke fluently.

Aidan was surprised to find among my books *Testament*, a collection of Tomi's anti-war cartoons from the late 1960s, early 1970s, bought in a remainder bookshop near the British Museum, and his account of the Nova Scotia farm, *Far Out Isn't Far Enough*. Aidan knew Tomi only as a writer of children's cartoon books, which his own sons had loved, and had not realised that he also wrote for adults. He immediately wanted to meet him. Yvonne invited us to lunch, and the two-hour drive to Dunlough in early summer became an annual ritual. It was apparent that Aidan's admiration for Tomi was reciprocated. On that first visit he gave Tomi a copy of a collection of his children's drawings and stories, *Colossal Congorr and the Turkes of Mars*, published in London by Jonathan Cape, and *Bornholm Night-Ferry*. In turn, we came away with armfuls of colourful books, each with a version of Tomi's elaborate signature and a hand-drawn cartoon. Tomi very much liked Aidan's cartoons and collages, and encouraged him in both.

Tomi was given to dramatic presentations of his current situation, battles with publishers, galleries, bureaucrats, politicians and increasingly his own health: recurring back problems followed by eye trouble. But he was also a good listener, and as well as asking Aidan what he was working on, always asked what I was up to. We usually spent some time with Tomi in the converted chapel that was his workroom, where he would talk about his current work projects, before eating a simple lunch with Yvonne, looking out over the

Mizen Head, often shrouded in mist. In spite of his aches and pains, Tomi overflowed with brilliant conversation. He often summed up the conclusion of his story in an aphorism; for example, 'If you respect food and nature, you cannot commit blasphemy.' I called these 'Ungerisms'. We told him, as had others before us, that he should publish a book of his aphorisms. In the year 2000, he presented us with exactly that, a book in French called Tomi Ungerer: *Vracs*.

Tomi, who was born in 1931, was writing a memoir of his childhood in wartime Alsace when he and Aidan first met. They shared an obsession with this period, and Aidan delighted in Tomi's childhood cartoons of Nazi-occupied Alsace, which his mother had kept. The review Aidan wrote when *Tomi – A Childhood Under the Nazis* appeared in a new English edition (1998) was one of his best. He prefaced it with one of his favourite Tomi quotes from the Nova Scotia book: 'After a spell on the dungpile went back to the studio to draw.' It was published in the *London Magazine* (sadly, it remains uncollected):

> This bittersweet account, pictorial and verbal, of Alsace during the Nazi occupation can be read as a sort of boy's version of the *Diary of Anne Frank*, but franker, fiercer, as behoves the hand that wrote it, drew it, with teeth clenched...
>
> 'My wife and butchery' Ungerer forcefully offered as his hobbies to one of those imbecile questionnaires to authors. 'The pigs I have drawn as an artist are pigs I have killed and butchered myself.'
>
> You can say that again. The art of butchering animals is akin to searing graphic work. Drawing and cutting up meat have a similar need for precision. What is cut cannot be uncut.[6]

Tomi usually left for Strasbourg in late summer, returning home in time for Christmas. It was his habit to ring around his friends to see how we were doing, and let us know he was back. The Tomi phone call was for many years part of our Christmas routine, a sign that the festive season had begun. I remember one in particular when he had come back to a house in need of much maintenance: 'I feel like a unicorn with a screwdriver on my head instead of a horn'. Tomi was the screwdriver man, and Yvonne, who has a strong rapport with animals, was the animal person. What I liked most about the Ungerers was the respect they had for each other's worlds. 'She has her business, and I have mine,' he said, watching lovingly as Yvonne, having spent the morning practising the piano, washed a batch of newly laid eggs. Yvonne listened quietly as Tomi dominated the table with his incessant stream of ideas sparking one off the other, chiming in occasionally, and was always listened to with respect. I wished that Aidan and I could share a similar harmony, instead of our rough-and-tumble way of rubbing along, which often deteriorated into arguments in front of guests. When I commented on this harmony to Aidan on the long drive home, he said it was not something he had noticed. But Yvonne recognised a familiar in me, another woman with a life of her own, striving to find a way to be the companion of a larger-than-life, dominant character who loved to hold the floor.

★

In 1988 Jill had published a novel about the break-up of their marriage in Berlin, *McDaid's Wife*.[7] It was a good, taut story, and well received. Aidan particularly liked the *Guardian*'s review, which referred to the husband figure (himself) as 'a drunken Irish poet of particularly goatish charm'.

Sometime later, Aidan remembered notebooks he had kept during the same era in Berlin. He asked Jill to send them from the Muswell Hill flat, where he had left them, and she did. There were two A4 notebooks, full of closely worked paragraphs, and a battered old school exercise book, the sort he used to buy in Ryman's in multipacks. This was held together by string passed through two holes made by a paper puncher. As usual he did not tell me what he was up to, but what he found in the notebooks was, essentially, a ready-made comic novel: *Lions of the Grunewald*. Aidan buckled down, lightly fictionalising the events in the diary, and wrote the novel in an extraordinary two and a half months. He worked at breakneck speed, often getting up as soon as he woke, even if it was still dark, and pounding away at the typewriter for two or three hours at a stretch. He would walk around Compass Hill at a cracking pace – in thirty minutes instead of the usual leisurely forty-five – take a short nap, and return to the typewriter, day after day.

Many of Aidan's admirers hold the novel in high esteem. It is a comic account of Professor Weaver's extra-marital affair, and the antics of his fellow writers in Berlin on the DAAD scholarship programme (fictionalised as DILDO).

I find the writing over-wrought and tiresome, and the characters too. To me, it is the least interesting of Aidan's fiction. Parts of the novel seem to have been written not by Aidan as I knew him, but by some monstruous alter ego, Aidan of the little devil who delights in boasting of his bad behaviour towards his wife. He even imagines her puzzling over his change of identity:

> Was this the same husband whom she had seen as kind and trustworthy? No paragon of virtue to be sure, but now he was the living embodiment of

duplicity, waywardness, lies. He was a congenital liar; a crafty manipulator, sneaky, shiftless, bone idle. He had no sense of … what was the word? Probity. He was one shifty schemer, economical with the truth; it was something he said when it suited him.[8]

Gerry Dukes in his *Irish Times* review sums it up neatly: 'The problem with the novel is that it reads as a series of set pieces which do not finally cohere … The locus of the problem is the character of Weaver, who rarely achieves higher levels of animation than that ascribed to him by his wife Nancy in her reference to his "over-active prick".'[9]

And yet this was the book that Tomi Ungerer loved the most. He once rang Aidan out of the blue, several years after it came out, to read to him over the phone the start of a chapter that he had found particularly amusing on rereading. Aidan was glowing for days after. Sometimes Tomi spoke of an illustrated edition, with his own cartoons of his favourite scenes.

★

In *The Importance of Being Earnest*, at the beginning of Act Two, which is set in the garden at the Manor House, Woolton, Miss Prism calls out to Cecily, who is watering the flowers: 'Cecily! Cecily! Surely such a utilitarian occupation as the watering of flowers is rather Moulton's duty than yours?'

In November 1993 we went to the play in Kinsale, which has an excellent theatre company, the Rampart Players. Aidan was especially taken with this character Moulton, who is such a small part of the play that he never even makes an appearance. He is there, offstage, to do menial tasks for the genteel young lady. He immediately appropriated Moulton's identity, and told me that would be his name in future: no more Squid. He was Moulton, there to do my bidding in house and garden. Moulton did the washing up, Moulton mowed the lawn, Moulton spent hours pulling ivy off the walls and weeds out of the paths. Moulton cleaned the ashes out of the wood-burning stove, carried turf briquettes and wood upstairs, Moulton did the Hoovering, he even, although out of character, did the ironing. Where would we be without Moulton?

*

For some time I had been encouraging Aidan to write an autobiography, covering those far-off years in Dublin after leaving school, hanging around with Arthur Power and Arland Ussher. I had listened to him exchanging memories of those days with George Morrison in 1988. It sounded fascinating, life as it could have been lived in Dublin any time in the earlier twentieth century, with regular salons, held on certain days of the week, and incompetent literary gents attempting to sail wooden boats at Dún Laoghaire in summer.

But instead Aidan went much further back, to his childhood and before, and wrote a very different, far more ambitious book, *Donkey's Years*. He was already mulling it over in his diary in November 1993, while correcting the proofs of *Lions of the Grunewald*: 'Zin's idea of autobiography – telling her of cycling from Howth to Greystones, soup at Powers'; Ussher and circle. Brother D in Largs, Brother Colman, Brother Brendan. A beginning already there. I was born 66 years ago in a big house called Springfield.'[10] Though we did not realise it at the time, it was to be the first of three volumes of memoirs. The 1990s were an extremely productive time for Aidan, and also included his seventieth birthday on 3 March 1997. In addition to the novel, *Lions of the Grunewald*, the memoirs, *Donkey's Years*, *Dog Days* and *The Whole Hog* (later published in one volume as *A Bestiary*), he also produced a text on Samuel Beckett to accompany John Minihan's photographs, and revised several of his short stories for inclusion in an expanded collection, *Flotsam and Jetsam*.

From the autumn of 1993 for the next six months or so, Aidan was thoroughly involved in the writing of *Donkey's Years*, reliving his childhood memories during long phone calls with Colman, and consulting Bernard Share on the local history of Celbridge and its characters. Bernard had lived for twelve years in his apartment in a wing of Springfield, and shared Aidan's obsessive interest with the past of the house.

Donkey's Years is subtitled *Memories of a Life as Story Told*, an apt description. This is, as he would say, the opening shot:

> I am consumed by memories and they form the life of me; stories that make up my life and lend it whatever veracity and purpose it may have. I suspect that even before I saw the light of day on 3rd March 1927 I was already being consumed by memories in Mumu's womb and by her memories prior to mine and by her granny's prior to her, bypassing my mother, stretching as far back as accommodating memory could reach into the past.

Donkey's Years is an extraordinary achievement, probably the best of all Aidan's books. He had at last found a theme (memory) and a mode (discursive autobiography) that suited his unique talents.*

He had never been entirely comfortable with the conventions of fiction writing ('The sullen art of fiction-writing can be a harrowing procedure; an inspired form of pillaging')[11], though in *Langrishe, Go Down* he showed himself well able to craft a memorable and atmospheric novel. *Scenes from a Receding Past* is a simpler exercise in the transformation of autobiographical material into a fictional form – a life lightly fictionalised. The more ambitious novel, *Balcony of Europe*, was originally intended as an experiment in writing a novel as it happened – an account of daily life as lived by the author rewritten as fiction. It was an interesting idea in theory, but it did not work in practice. While there are wonderful set-pieces, wonderful descriptive passages and much memorable writing about sexual obsession, it simply does not cohere. But when he takes his own experiences as the theme, and his earliest memories as a starting point for an autobiography that will have its own logic and its own rules, he is in the right place for his ability as a writer to shine through. And because he knew that he was at last on the right track, he declared (in an Appendix) that *Scenes* and *Balcony* would remain out of print for the rest of his life: 'I have freely pillaged from both for sections of this present work – bold Robin Crusoe ferrying booty from two wrecks.'

I think that the genesis of *Donkey's Years* lies partly in the piece he wrote in 1986 about Athy for the magazine *Cara*,[12] that

---

* The dust jacket of *Donkey's Years* features an especially charming photograph of Aidan aged about six, standing in the shrubbery with his hand on the cap of a garden gnome. It will be familiar to readers of the Calder hardback of *Scenes from a Receding Past* (1977), where it was also featured on the dust jacket.

was edited by Bernard Share, to accompany John Minihan's photographs of the wake of Katie Tyrrell. He spent at least one night in Athy, at that time a run-down backwater in rural Kildare, where the physical surroundings took him right back to his childhood. Bernard Share recalls that the piece almost got him fired, and quotes from a letter Aidan sent him with the piece: 'A mood piece I hope or trust not too leery, because the place itself was and is DESPERATE. Had quite forgot what a miserable place Kildare can be.'[13] The piece is a tour de force of memory, as one thing seemed to lead to another, and also a hymn of praise to the unique charms of County Kildare. Parts of it were adapted and personalised by the inclusion of Mumu and Dado and Sister Rumold, and incorporated into the opening chapter of *Donkey's Years*, beginning:

> When did you last see a woman wringing her hands or an old fellow wearing vulcanite bicycle clips or nervous black greyhounds on the leash or the inextinguishable fires of wayside itinerants and their washing draped on hedges and bushes and they themselves (The Great Unwashed) none too clean?[14]

Another chance to immerse himself in memories of Kildare came when Robin Robertson commissioned him to write the Kildare text for the collection of photographs by Donovan Wylie, *32 Counties*, with an essay about each county by thirty-two Irish writers. Aidan had a deep affection for his home county; on the Cork–Dublin train he would always know when we had crossed the county boundary into Kildare, by a subtle change of light, the hugeness of the sky, 'the piling-up of brilliantly white cirro-cumulus, the frisky air of the Liffey valley'.

His piece on Kildare for *32 Counties* begins:

I remember it in the time of paraffin lamps, anthracite, sago, Bird's Custard, farthings, wetted coke, servants, triple-layer buns from Boland's delivery van, frog-spawn and tadpoles wriggling in the pond at the edge of the Crooked Meadow....[15]

This has also been spruced up and incorporated into the first chapter of *Donkey's Years*.

But more importantly, three chapters from Part One of *Balcony of Europe* in which his mother's death is described slowly in precise moving detail, have been incorporated into *Donkey's Years* towards the end. The vividly evoked childhood incidents from *Scenes from a Receding Past*, Mumu teaching Aidan to read, for example, are similarly incorporated. As Colm Tóibín wrote in 1996: 'In Aidan Higgins's worlds, things are allowed to happen three times, first real, then fiction, then real again.'[16] And why not?

But no knowledge of all this pillaging and plundering is needed to enjoy the autobiography. The main section, about two-thirds of the book, is an account of Aidan's childhood in Kildare, his schooldays at Killashee and Clongowes (a chapter entitled 'The Bracing Air of Sodom'), the move from the splendour of Springfield to a small bungalow in Greystones, and his first job away from home as a golfing partner to an ailing alcoholic on the Isle of Man (already written as fiction in 'Asylum').

It is the energy of the writing, its detail and its unpredictable changes of direction and tone of voice that hold the reader's interest. The skinny child, the faddy eater, is cast into misery taking literally servant Lizzy Bolger's throwaway remark, 'Yewer Mammy's run off with a sailor.' He haunts the kitchen, listening to the tales of the butcher's boy, the Bowsy

Murray, 'a strong, stumpy little man', with an intensity that gives the skinny child the superhuman strength to topple the kitchen table over. The close bond with his trusting younger brother Colman/Colum, rechristened 'the Dote', is evident in the description of their childish games, while his dislike of his eldest brother, 'the Dodo', is overwhelming:

> I hide under the long table in the diningroom. The linen cloth reaches to the floor, and my patience with my elder brother is exhausted. I wait until the family have taken their places and then growling like a mad dog sink my teeth into the white calf of brother Dodo's leg and hang on as he rises straight up with a high-pitched scream. I taste pure venom in my mouth as he staggers from the room.[17]

Part Two consists of a section on his working life in London, and his meeting with Jill Anders, who is to become his wife, before the journey to Africa with John Wright's Marionette Theatre described in Part Three. The final section recounts his homecoming with wife and baby, and continues with a memorably poignant description of his mother's death in Dún Laoghaire.

Donkey's Years was the first book that Aidan worked on with Geoff Mulligan as editor. A good-humoured man originally from Belfast, he had taken over when Robin Robertson left Secker for Jonathan Cape. He let Aidan work away with it, with a minimum of interference, and consequently he and Aidan got on well. Geoff was also Roddy Doyle's editor.

The memoir was well received, though Derek Mahon, writing a retrospective overview of Aidan's work in 2007 (after the publication of all three volumes of memoirs in one book as *A Bestiary*) claims that the memoirs received less attention than they deserved on first publication, and that there was often a hostile note in those reviews that did appear: 'He can be expressionist and baroque, lyrical and grotesque, fastidious and colloquial by turns, and presumes a like-minded "browser" of comparable erudition and unsentimentality. His whole practice and attitude are about as far as one could get from current aesthetics, though it would be wrong to think of him as conservative. Not at all: he is, paradoxically, the most blithely subversive of writers…'[18]

Perhaps the most telling short endorsement of *Donkey's Years* is Dermot Healy's: 'Leaving down *Donkey's Years* at four in the morning after one straight reading I felt exhilarated …. Read it and see. Few books inspire like this.'

*

Due more to circumstances than ambition, I started working as an art critic. I was already writing arts features for the *Irish Examiner* when their reviewer of art moved to Dublin, so I stepped in. This was the start of a boom in contemporary Irish art that lasted until the crash of 2008. I was able to cover the main Dublin openings and also the Venice Biennale, and some of the London shows. For a few years I was also Dublin theatre critic for the *Financial Times* (their new theatre critic did not fly), which involved overnight trips to Dublin every six weeks or so, writing the review next morning on the train home. The money for writing about art wasn't that good, but I enjoyed the travel, the people involved were usually interesting, and the occasional excursions fitted in well with the rest of my life. The *Sunday Times* started an Irish edition, and I volunteered to cover arts in the south-west for them. Then the *Irish Arts*

Review, a glossy magazine, went from one edition a year to four, and gave me regular work.

Summer was a busy time in the south-west, and I enjoyed the well-attended openings, as did Aidan, who often came along. The London gallerist Angela Flowers had a holiday home in Rosscarbery, about an hour west of Kinsale, where she held an annual show of new work. Another twenty kilometres further west, Margaret Warren, a generous patron of the arts from Texas, had established a gallery in a restored boathouse in Castletownshend, a quiet seaside village with a cluster of 'big houses', and had at least one show a year, usually curated by Peter Murray. There was definitely a whiff of glamour about these occasions, especially when the sun shone. One time Aidan introduced himself to a tall, grey-haired man with a book bag on his shoulder, assuming, correctly, that he would be a keen reader, and therefore interesting to talk to. He was Greg Schirmer, an academic originally from Chicago, currently teaching in Oxford, Mississippi, who fled the heat of the deep south to spend summers in west Cork with his wife, Jane Mullen. Jane had published a collection of stories, and was working on a historical novel set in west Cork. Greg's academic area was Irish poetry in the English language. He was a good friend of Eudora Welty, whose work Aidan revered, while Richard Ford admired Jane's work. The four of us met regularly every summer for many years.

Much as I enjoyed the art world, I had not given up writing fiction. I still had hopes that the historical novel would find a publisher. I also usually finished a few short stories in the course of a year, and occasionally published one in the *London Magazine* and other small reviews. But as there was very little money in publishing stories, I gave story-writing a low priority. I had tried for several years placing stories with David Marcus, who edited an annual publication of the best Irish stories, but they were consistently rejected. Eventually a letter scrawled by hand arrived saying 'Please desist from submitting stories to me. Your work belongs in the better type of woman's magazine.'

★

In May 1994, with *Donkey's Years* nearing completion, Geoff Mulligan contacted Aidan to say that Secker were going to publish John Minihan's photographs of Samuel Beckett, and that he and John had agreed that Aidan would be the ideal person to write a text to accompany them. Aidan had already worked with John Minihan, having written about his hometown of Athy in County Kildare to accompany the photographic essay in *Cara* magazine. John was one of several people that Aidan and I knew separately before we met. He had been a colleague of mine in London at the *Evening Standard* before moving to west Cork with his young family.

Aidan did not seem inclined to accept the Beckett commission. I had assumed he would be thrilled: there was a generous fee, and he knew and liked the photos. But it would also involve hard work. Beckett is difficult to write about at the best of times, but given Aidan's deep admiration of his work and his intelligence, it must have been daunting. People and places you feel deeply about are always the most difficult to write about.

'Well,' I said, seeing a way of motivating him, 'if you don't do it, they'll probably ask John Montague.'

'How do you know?'

'It's obvious. He's the next in line. He's full of opinions, and he's always boasting about what good friends he and Beckett were. And if not him, then Anthony Cronin.'

Aidan had always doubted John Montague's claims to be a regular drinking pal of Beckett's in Paris, but why would the poet lie? Unlike Aidan, Montague had lived in Paris for extended periods, and spoke excellent French. And Aidan had a highly competitive relationship with his old friend Anthony Cronin, who was in fact working on his biography of Beckett at the time.

My bluff worked, for that is what it was. I had no idea who Secker would ask if Aidan said no. Montague was only a guess, and so was Cronin, but the suggestion paid off. Aidan immediately contacted Geoff and accepted the commission.

Aidan's friendship with Beckett had mainly been conducted by letters, which are now in the collection of the Harry Ransom Center in Austin, Texas. They had met maybe half a dozen times, in London, Paris and Berlin. The last meeting was in Berlin in 1969, where Beckett was rehearsing *Krapp's Last Tape*.

Anthony Cronin, in his biography of Beckett, reports Aidan's reaction to that Berlin meeting:

> He found Beckett's politeness almost intolerable and the inhibition about saying anything about his work devastating, so that one wound up feeling that it would be better not to say anything at all; but with the resulting silence came a sense of painful inadequacy.[19]

Cronin mentions Aidan's contribution to *Beckett at Sixty: A Festschrift*[20] as possibly being a key to the cooling of the friendship. Aidan's 'Tribute' consisted of a less than enthusiastic description of Beckett's *How It Is* (1964):

No Celia, nor Moran, no Watt, no light, no cockle, no vetch, only mud, a mud of words ... coldness and reason. Worlds once, now only words, uncharted places. Into this thin mist of words the most accomplished master of English prose since Joyce is disappearing.

He restates this more clearly in a piece published by his old friend John Ryan in 1970:

> *Malone Dies* and *Molloy* are written with a clarity and bile that recall Swift. But already apparent in the latter is the 'balls-aching boredom' with fictional themes that was to blight his later fiction like a disease in trees. I confess that I cannot follow him into *The Unnamable*, much less beyond it into *How It Is*. These astringent philosophical works are beyond the patience of most.[21]

It looks to me quite simply a case of the protégé outgrowing the mentor, two writers with busy lives, and in Beckett's case a heavy burden of correspondence, naturally growing apart. This estrangement has absolutely nothing to do with Beckett calling *Langrishe* 'literary shit' at a party in 1966, an anecdote that Aidan loved to tell and retell, in print and in person. In his version his wife Jill presses Beckett for an opinion of the new novel, while Beckett demurs, saying that he hasn't finished it. Eventually, pressed again for a comment, he snaps, 'Literary shit'.

In mid-September Geoff decided to come to Kinsale to work on the editing of the Beckett piece with Aidan. Usually this was done by post, typescripts going to and fro, and phone calls.

So far, while working on the first volume of memoirs, Geoff had proved to be a very light-handed editor, open to Aidan's unusual ways. We organised a room for him with our friend Jimmie Conron, whose friendly B&B was effectively our 'spare room'. We booked a table for dinner at a nearby country house hotel, which would be quieter than Kinsale, still busy with tourists. We picked Geoff up at the airport and drove to an old-fashioned country pub right on the river at Kilmacsimon Quay, a picturesque spot. It was high tide on a limpid early autumn evening, the trees just starting to turn, and we all relaxed.

I was working on a new draft of the west Cork eighteenth-century novel, firmly believing that there was a publisher for it somewhere. Reg had effectively retired due to ill health, and I was looking for a new agent. Geoff said he had a friend, also from Belfast, who might be interested in taking me on, which cheered me up greatly.

Back in Kinsale we retreated to our local – and Jimmie's – the Tap Tavern, where Jimmie was playing mandolin, and singing ballads. The arrival of the crew of the *Asgard* – including Tim Goulding's wife Annie from Allihies – and their gregarious skipper Tom McCarthy, an old sailing pal of mine, put an end to any further conversation, but provided some memorable entertainment.

The next morning Aidan and Geoff were up by nine, working at his desk. I made them coffee and sandwiches so that they could work straight through until 3 p.m., when Geoff was collected by a pre-ordered car. After an oddly formal handshake at the front door, he was off to the airport. It may have been formal, but there had been no major disagreements and absolutely no lingering resentment on Aidan's part. He seemed well pleased. We went straight out for a long walk toward the west, and home along the river again to an early night.

I read the Beckett piece again just now, after many years, and I understand why Geoff thought it worth the effort to come to Kinsale and work on it face to face. It is a terrific piece, Aidan at his best, but also Aidan at his most elliptical and mischievous. Goodness knows what sort of shape it was in before the edit. Even after editing, there are times when it teeters on the brink of being hijacked by one or other of Aidan's obsessions, but then its sails are trimmed, and it goes back on its rightful course. As Aidan puts it in the fourth sentence: 'Sam Beckett, that *Terra incognita* ever receding, was never an easy subject to entrap.'

He puts Beckett in the context of early twentieth-century Ireland, emerging from 'a Celtic mist', into the dead place that was Dublin in the 1930s and 1940s. Only after *Watt* (his last text in English, dismissed by its author as 'execrable'), and the *Trilogy*, written in French and never, according to its author, satisfactorily translated into English, did Beckett find his *modus operandi*:

> Joyce's archetypal mummies were superseded by Beckett's retarded and half-witted, men and women come down in the world, in a narrative fuelled by Godlike (or Godot-like) uncertainty and doubt.
>
> Where now? Who now? When now?
>
> 'Next to great joy,' rumbled clubman Henry James, pulling on a thick cigar, 'no state of mind is so frolicsome as great distress.'[22]

Proceeding in a vertiginously intuitive manner, the next section traces Beckett's antecedents – James Joyce (without ever mentioning the fact that Beckett was for several years

Joyce's secretary and amanuensis) and his fellow Protestant, Elizabeth Bowen.

In Part Three Myles na gCopaleen, Brian O'Nolan and briefly Flann O'Brien all have a part to play, referencing his elders, Beckett and Joyce, and leading Aidan to bring himself into the proceedings for the first time:

> Brian O'Nolan, the speaker of Tyrone Gaelic, would pay grudging homage to Joyce, but in the next breath would have to disparage him, and to Beckett of all people who would in turn refuse to read *At Swim-Two-Birds* because of the imagined slight to Joyce, and would in turn tell it to me in the Giraffe Restaurant in Klopstockstrasse in Berlin. 'Joyce,' spat out Myles the begrudger, 'that refurbisher of skivvies' stories!' It may have gone down well as a public sally in the Scotch House or acid aside in the Pearl Bar, but it didn't go down well with Beckett, deviser of the voice and of its hearer and of himself, most certainly not.[23]

Having broken the ice, Aidan continues to draw on his own experience of Beckett:

> I once asked Beckett his opinion on Joyce (the awe-tist *ne plus ultra*, not the man), in one word. He didn't hesitate: 'Probity,' said Sam stoutly. I've heard it defined as a ferocious application to the task in hand.[24]

After a comparison of *Gulliver's Travels*, *Murphy* and *At Swim-Two-Birds* as satires of the Irish psyche, Aidan finds one thing the two twentieth-century writers had in common: 'Both Beckett and O'Nolan had independently admitted to me that they could see no virtue in their first novels.'[25]

He was not apparently tempted to bring himself into the picture, even though as a writer he is often cited as someone who never wrote a better novel than his first, *Langrishe, Go Down*.

Until the obituaries that followed his death in 1989, many readers were not aware of the close connection between Beckett's activities in the French Resistance and his post-war work, *Godot* in particular, and Aidan covers this well. For all the intellectual flights and friskiness of Aidan's attempts to place Beckett within the pantheon of twentieth-century Irish writers, probably the most memorable aspects of this piece are Aidan's own memories of the times he spent with Sam. He points out that this most austere of men was capable of warm friendships with a wide variety of people, including certain actors, who had an intuitive understanding of what he was after:

> Despite his frigid bearing and frosty mien, there was something warm and endearing about him. Few if any ever called him Samuel; it was always Sam. If he liked you, well and good, you were instantly accepted into the closed circle, the enclave. He gave with an open hand and had to be taken with the same reciprocal spirit, as unstintingly. Was it this that inspired affection, or was it his work, so affecting, or was it a combination of both? One was privileged to know Sam Beckett, for his likes will not come again: such generosity of spirit was rarer than radium.[26]

*

In October 1994, Derek and Aidan were both invited to read at the Harbourfront Writers' Festival in Toronto. Derek was living in New York in Greenwich Village, a couple of blocks from the Tenth Street Pier. His friend Patricia King was working at the Glucksman Ireland House, part of New York University, located in an elegant town house just off Washington Square. The Harbourfront people offered accommodation to any 'spouses' who wanted to attend the festival, but not travel. Derek decided that if we were going to Toronto, we should also visit New York, and arranged for Aidan to be invited to give a paper at Ireland House. We would stay the first weekend in Patricia King's apartment, at her invitation, and NYU would give us accommodation at Union Square from Monday to Friday, plus a fee for Aidan. The only expense would be my return fare, which was do-able.

A break before the long Irish winter was very welcome. We arrived at Ireland House around 5 p.m. on a Friday, after a classic taxi ride from JFK across the 59th Street Bridge in bright autumn sunshine. Our Afghan taxi driver had never heard of Washington Square *Mews*, but we found it with no trouble. There was a film crew outside, and someone hushed us while we paid our driver, as a loud voice-over proclaimed: 'This broadcast comes to you courtesy of the America-Ireland Fund.'

We left our cases at Pat's place, which was under the eaves of another tall town house in the mews. Aidan declared it to be ten storeys up – it was of course only five, with two flights of stairs per floor. Edward Hopper had his studio in this building, we were told. Derek was in big-city mode in a smart seersucker suit, and whisked us off to his favourite restaurant, the Knickerbocker, for a celebratory dinner, along with his friend Seamus Deane. Pat, as was her custom, went home to Connecticut for the weekend.

The Knickerbocker Bar and Grill is a Greenwich Village institution, an old-fashioned restaurant with the air of a

Bohemian gentleman's dining club, with wood-panelled walls, mahogany and brass fittings, and framed posters of American memorabilia from the early twentieth century. The waiters were mainly moonlighting actors, and recited long lists of daily specials with dramatic brio. Aidan immediately felt at home. Modern jazz was playing quietly in the background: no bland pop music in the Knickerbocker. He was advised to order crab cakes, a novelty to us, and for once he was well-pleased with his plate. I got the impression from Derek that the Knickerbocker was a place kept for special occasions. To us, used only to Irish restaurant prices, it did not seem expensive.

I was up early and walked around Washington Square in the glorious autumn sunlight before collecting Aidan, and meeting Derek at his chosen diner. He was carrying *A Literary Guide to New York*, and I had bought a good map of Manhattan. Our first stop was Patchin Place, a historic cul-de-sac not far from 10th Street where Djuna Barnes had lived for the last forty years of her life. She liked to describe this as her 'Trappist' period. It was a strange old building in a narrow, gated alley with iron balconies and fire escapes on the building's front giving access to the apartments. Aidan told us that e. e. cummings had an apartment in the same building. Every so often he would throw open his window and holler 'Are ya still alive, Djuna?' We took a cab to Strand Books, probably the only place in New York where we could find copies of our own work. Aidan bought *Bornholm Night-Ferry* and my first novel, *A Joke Goes a Long Way in the Country*, as a present for Pat. I bought half a dozen books by and about Edith Wharton that were not in print in the UK, intending to post them home. Tired after the journey and the excitement of arrival, we spent Saturday night in, watching a golf tournament on TV. I was starting to realise that one of the reasons we did not have television at home was that, if it was there, Aidan would not be able to resist the temptation to watch it. At last I had an explanation for his unusually deep knowledge of the characters in *Glenroe*: he must have been a regular viewer in the cottage in Wicklow.

We were up early on the Sunday, kept awake by street noise and drums being beaten in Washington Square. Because the weather was so good we walked down to Battery Point through eerily empty streets, past the World Trade Center and its tall towers, which were new since my last visit to New York. It was cloudy but warm, and we got the first boat out to Ellis Island, with a photo stop at the Statue of Liberty. In the main hall we looked up the computer covering the years 1880–1924 and found both Higginses and Scanlons (my Kerry grandmother's family) among the early immigrants. Tom Higgins, from whom Aidan's father inherited the money that enabled him to buy Springfield, emigrated to Bisbee, Arizona, where he made his fortune first with a copper mine and then in property development in California.

We were both struck by the speed with which a human drama becomes history and then a $6 tourist attraction. We were also by impressed by the beauty of the recently restored buildings, in contrast to the many sad stories that had been enacted there. We were both especially curious about those who didn't make the grade, and were denied entry to the USA on grounds of bad health – usually TB. Aidan later incorporated a reference to this excursion into his paper:

> I was out the other morning on the ferry to Ellis Island
> to look over the ethnic museum you have there, the
> chamber of horrors; to see the rites of passage that
> admitted or didn't admit immigrants into the Land

of the Free – a rite of passage as painful as birth pangs that become death pangs for some unfortunates who never made the grade, were refused admission.[27]

Because the weather was so pleasant and the streets traffic-free, we walked back uptown, eventually taking a cab up to Union Square, where we had been recommended a place for brunch. Aidan refused to contemplate the subway system, so I did not insist. We were only here for a few days, and if he wanted to go everywhere by cab, why not? Time to drop the old habits from student days. So next morning we took a taxi to the Guggenheim Museum. The driver warned us that the Columbus Day parade on Fifth Avenue was causing traffic problems. Aidan was always totally absorbed in a gallery once he liked what was on show, and he was well-pleased by a special exhibition with major works by Cézanne, Gauguin and Picasso. He especially liked Picasso's *The Lobster and the Cat*. But he was in a strange mood, and I couldn't work out what was bothering him. He kept snapping at me for no particular reason, accused me of disappearing, of walking too slowly, walking too fast, objecting when I stopped him jay-walking. It was a relief to stand on Fifth Avenue for a few minutes watching the marching bands of the NYPD and the baton-twirlers from the local high schools. Having suddenly had enough, Aidan walked me around the corner, where he summoned a taxi to the Knickerbocker for lunch. When I suggested we might try somewhere else, he said why bother, when you knew you would get a good meal at the Knickerbocker?

I was glad when we finally checked in to our new NYU apartment. I wasn't feeling well, either fighting off a sore throat or reacting badly to the air of New York, and was glad to dose myself with remedies from the drugstore and have a rest.

Derek was teaching that night, and suggested we try Pete's Tavern near Gramercy Park, a traditional bar, but it was busy when we got there, and there were no seats. We had noticed that Alice Munro was reading at the 92nd Street Y with Carol Shields, so we took a cab up to the Y. We had a couple of hours to kill, so Aidan asked the woman selling tickets where we could find a decent bar nearby. She mentioned the Kinsale Tavern as being the best bet and, even though it was a sports bar, she said we should find a quiet corner. The coincidence of the name cheered us both up.

The reading was packed. It was interesting to see this place that was so often advertised in the *New York Review of Books*, and to get an idea of its large scale. We didn't know Carol Shields' work and were not expecting much, but she was very good. And Alice Munro was extraordinary, a slight woman, very thin, who read with an unusual intensity from a new story called 'The Albanian Virgin' for almost an hour. It was as if the person in front of us had disappeared, and all that remained was the disembodied story. There was a wine reception afterwards, and we bought a copy of her new book, *Friend of My Youth*. Aidan eventually joined the queue to get our book signed. He had been exchanging letters with Alice, fan letters, and he was deliberately the last in the queue, hoping to have a chat once his turn came. I was fading, between the long day and the sore throat, and took a seat nearby and dozed. Eventually I was awoken by a loud shout of 'Rory of the Hills!' Aidan had identified himself, and Alice was thrilled. She was also exhausted, and after a short but very amiable chat, we left for our new quarters in Union Square.

The next day, Tuesday, was the day of Aidan's reading at Ireland House. There would be a dinner after for about sixteen of us at the Knickerbocker. It was obviously Ireland

House's staff canteen. I left Aidan alone for the morning in our dark, functional apartment, which seemed to be full of sharp edges and elusive light switches. I walked up to the luxury department store Barney's, which my sister had told me I must see. It was nice, but impossibly expensive. I bought some music cassettes at Goody's, and enjoyed being out on my own, with nobody sniping at my heels.

Aidan had arranged to meet Mike Heller, a poet he had known in Nerja in the 1960s, at the Knickerbocker for lunch. He was still earning his living by teaching English as a foreign language, thirty years after returning from Spain, which seemed a bit sad to me. He had of course known Jill in Nerja, and I quickly realised he was not interested in talking to me, only Aidan. Fair enough.

We went back to our apartment to change for the big event. Derek was introducing Aidan, so he left first as he had arranged to meet him at – yes, the Knickerbocker, the only place he knew how to find on his own. I arrived just after them at Ireland House, where a good crowd was gathering. I was getting used to public readings now, and Aidan was far more confident of being able to hold the floor: he was starting to enjoy entertaining an audience. This was the best reading he had given so far, in a beautiful first-floor drawing room, a full forty minutes, followed by warm applause. There was a reception downstairs afterwards. Aidan had been wanting to meet Barney Rosset, who had published Beckett in the States and worked closely with John Calder, and there he was, with his wife Astrid, Mike Heller and his wife, an English agent who was looking after Aidan's work in New York for Secker, and Sharon Ames, a lively woman about my age, a voracious reader, whom we had met recently in Kinsale. When she said, 'Look me up if you're ever in New York,' we never thought we would be.

Pat had taken the next day off, and accompanied by Derek, his *Guide to Literary New York*, and some photocopies, drove us out to Cornwall-on-Hudson, Djuna Barnes's birthplace. Pat did indeed look tired, but seemed to recover in the course of the day. I was in heaven: there are few things I like more than being driven around a strange place, and shown interesting things. It was another sunny blue day, and as we drove up the West Side and over George Washington Bridge on to Palisades Parkway and Westpoint, all these names familiar from novels and stories – Cheever, Updike, Edith Wharton – suddenly took on a physical form. The Hudson River was even more impressive than I had expected. Cornwall was in Fall colours, the leaves blazing flame-red, orange and purple. Derek said the river was as magnificent as the Danube. It was a regular shingle-and-picket-fence New England town, spruced up with white paint, and as charming as you could wish for.

We had lunch at the Painters Tavern, which seemed to be the kind of place where the bank manager and the town lawyer would take their midday meal. But there was nothing specific in the guidebook about where Djuna Barnes grew up. We had a photocopy of the place where her ashes had been scattered, and a less clear one of her birthplace, labelled only 'Storm King Mountain'. Derek had the good idea of going to the post office to buy some stamps, guessing that if anyone had a lead on the birthplace of the town's most famous daughter, it would be the postmistress. He was right: she sent us to the library, where the town historian, Janet Dempsey, was at work in the basement. She was less than enthusiastic, and told us frostily that not much was known in Cornwall about the Barnes family. It seems they were from 'out of town'. She said to Pat in an aside, 'They were not respectable you know, the family.' We drove up and around Storm King Mountain with our photocopies, speculating about which of the elaborate remodelled chalets could be the one in the picture. There was no obvious candidate. But we did find the house in our other photocopy, the one with a dogwood grove behind it, in which her ashes were scattered.

It had been a long day, and I envied Pat going back alone to her cosy attic apartment. Derek wanted to take Aidan to the Lion's Head, an old-fashioned writers' pub in the Village that had been his local when he was drinking. He left us at the door, and went on home. We were hungry, so we ordered some food, lasagne, and for once I had to agree with Aidan's verdict: 'inedible'. But I ate enough to keep me going, hoping to head back for an early night. I was not best pleased when Aidan insisted on another cab ride to the Knickerbocker, where he ordered crab cakes in the bar while I, sore throat raging, sipped water. Because it was his first trip to New York, I didn't want to ruin it by being ill, but I was feeling terrible, and would have appreciated some allowance being made for that. But he hardly seemed to notice, so absorbed was he in his own pleasure.

I hardly slept a wink, between the sore throat, the cough and the garbage trucks congregating outside our windows at 6 a.m. Sharon Ames had invited us out to her house in East Hampton, as she had to drive up there the next day, and knew that Aidan was keen to visit Montauk nearby. Aidan agreed, so I rang her, and she said she'd pick us up at five. He had recently read Max Frisch's strange book of that name, and had questioned Sharon about the place while she was in Kinsale. After the usual diner breakfast, we spent the morning in the Met, where there was a superb Impressionist exhibition. We had to return a book to Pat at Ireland House and say goodbye. She passed on compliments on his paper from her boss. We still had time to pass before being picked up for the drive to East Hampton. And where else to spend it but the Knickerbocker? At least we were within walking distance. We sat in the bar, me with a Coke, and Aidan with a last Martini. I made some remark, but Aidan didn't hear me. He was staring fixedly at a distinguished-looking middle-aged man up at the bar, also drinking a Martini. The man at the bar ordered another, and a bowl of soup. I repeated what I had said, and was shushed, and flicked away with a bad-tempered gesture. He was as if in a different world, where I didn't exist, or didn't matter, still staring at the two Martinis and a bowl of soup man. He shut me out. I was nothing to him, an irrelevance. Then he stood up and walked across the bar, holding out his hand to the stranger, as if to introduce himself: 'Denis O'Donoghue? Aidan Higgins.'

'Donoghue, no "O"' was the testy reply, but he did at least shake the proffered hand.

'I read you in the *New York Review of Books*.'

'Do you indeed?'

'Barney Rosset told me you had lunch here every day: two Martinis and a bowl of soup.'

A friend in common having been established, the conversation between the two men could proceed. I sat alone with my Coke, wondering who this person was who had shushed me so dismissively and introduced himself to a stranger in such an ingratiating way. It was not the Aidan I knew. He had never spoken to me like that before, nor had he ever spoken to another person in such a fawning tone. I knew at that moment that my feelings for him and his for me would never be the same again. There was a sliver of ice between us where none had been before. The honeymoon was over.

It had lasted eight years, almost to the day.

★

We got home on a Saturday, and it was a pleasure to wake up the next day in our own bed, sunlight streaming in the window. We had enjoyed our night in East Hampton and a takeout breakfast on the beach at Montauk; Toronto had gone well too, a huge, well-organised festival, with luxurious accommodation on the twenty-ninth floor of a waterfront hotel, and a roster of international writers coming and going, including our friend Derek Mahon. But the travel and the relentless socialising, and in Aidan's case two major public readings and one public 'conversation', had left us exhausted. The house looked small, shabby and untidy, and the hall needed painting. The mail consisted mostly of press releases for me.

We started bickering that Sunday, and stayed like that for several months. He told me that my voice had changed since getting back, become cowed, and I told him that his voice had an unpleasant crossness in it that had not been there before the trip.

Aidan had been up since 4 a.m. writing a letter to the *Irish Times* about Gerry Adams and the peace process, which hinged on a not-very-good *double entendre* involving peacemakers and two kinds of pacemakers. I had more faith in Gerry Adams than he did, but didn't want to get into a major row, so I didn't make any comment. Was this the new Aidan? If so, I didn't like him. The weather was changeable, rain-sun. I hung the washing out in light rain, feeling foolish and confused, hoping sun would follow.

Suddenly, all concern, Aidan realised how busy I'd been since we got back, unpacking, washing clothes, cleaning the house and food shopping, and suggested we go out to lunch so that, 'You do not have to lift a finger'. Then he ticked me off for driving too fast before we had even got into the car. In the restaurant, he talked to everyone, including the waiters, querying their nationality. Luckily, we were late by Irish Sunday lunch times, and only two other tables were taken. On our way home he was keen to drop in on our friends Katherine and Joachim to go on talking, but I insisted on driving straight home.

I had already recognised in Toronto that he was what I called 'hyper' – something that happened from time to time, a high, a kind of over-excitement combined with inexhaustible energy, but never had it been so extreme.

★

That spring there was a lunch party at the Simpsons to celebrate the publication of *Donkey's Years*. A trestle table was laid for sixteen people in Howard's study, a converted dry-stone barn. There was a gang of us known as 'the usual suspects' – Katherine and Joachim, Gerry and Marcia, Peter Murray and Sarah Iremonger, all lively company with strong opinions, and lovers of good food and wine. The Simpsons always served light, tasty food, often Mediterranean or Vietnamese in origin. Aidan had prepared a small speech – which he always called 'an address' – in which he reminded us all that from now on he would like to be known as 'Rory', short for 'Rory of the Hills', the character he had invented as the narrator of *Donkey's Years*. He explained that once he had decided to call himself Rory, his mother 'Mumu', his father 'Dado' and brother Colman 'the Dote', the book had practically written itself. A toast was proposed by Howard to Rory of the Hills.

About a year later, soon after *Donkey's Years* had come out in paperback, there was another lunch at the Simpsons', a smaller one, with the usual suspects again. Howard had a habit of carrying the latest review of his most recent book in the top inner pocket of his jacket, and would take other writers aside, and let you read it – whether it was a serious work of military history with an introduction by Pierre Salinger, or his latest pot-boiler about the wily French detective, Bastide. I found this habit very endearing, and enjoyed being included in this harmless shop-talk. Aidan, who otherwise liked Howard very much, hated it, and saw it as Howard showing off and asking for praise.

There was a general rule at the Simpsons' that you did not sit next to your spouse. I was so involved with my corner of the table that I didn't notice who Aidan was sitting with, but assumed that he was having as good a time as I was. But as people started to leave, I noticed that Aidan was no longer there. I looked around outside in case he had stepped out for a cigar, which Howard sometimes gave him, but no sign. I guessed that he must have walked home on his own, as he did occasionally when a party went on too long for his liking. But I was surprised that he had not said a quiet goodbye to one of our hosts. Such bad manners were unusual in Aidan. When I got home, he was in bed, but not yet asleep.

'What happened? Didn't you enjoy the party?'

'Didn't you notice?'

'Notice what?'

'All that they talked about was *Angela's Ashes*. Nobody mentioned *Donkey's Years*. Not once.'

There had indeed been an animated conversation about Frank McCourt's 'misery memoir', the story of his impoverished family life in Brooklyn and Limerick City. It was published the year after *Donkey's Years*. Most of us had read it, and nobody had liked it, considering it sentimental and over-the-top. But neither did anyone think to compare McCourt's relatively straightforward, tear-jerking memoir with Aidan's far more highly wrought volume.

McCourt's book was a bestseller, and won the 1996 National Book Critics' Circle Award for Biography, and the 1997 Pulitzer Prize for biography. The film, co-written and directed by Alan Parker, was released in 1999, and took $13 million at the box office. Another world.

Aidan had one more problem with *Donkey's Years*: it had not been reviewed by the *London Review of Books*. Nor had they reviewed *Lions of the Grunewald*, two years earlier. Derek, who was now living in Dublin, did his best to find out what was going on, and volunteered to write an overview himself if one was not already in train. He wrote to Aidan:

> *The LRB now tell me Donkey's Years has in fact been sent for review (they won't say to whom), and the sort of Higgins overview piece I'd envisaged will indeed appear. Their nameless reviewer is expected to write also about Ronda Gorge and Lions, since they didn't review those when they first came out. All this from John Lanchester, asst. ed., since Mary K. W. is now on holiday. I think she must have got some wires crossed before she left. In any case, expect soon a substantial LRB essay: my guess is sometime in September.*[28]

It never appeared.

★

A photograph on the noticeboard in our local supermarket caught my eye – five gorgeous little black kittens, and beside it a postcard with the words 'Free to Good Homes'. I took a note of the number, and it turned out to belong our friends Horace and Phyllis Lysaght. Such coincidences were not unusual in a small town like Kinsale. Horace was planning to take early retirement from his job as a bank manager, and move to Nerja to paint. Meanwhile they had bult a house on the Bandon River in a place called Sleepy Hollow, above a shingle beach said to be frequented by otters. The mother cat, Chloe, was a real beauty, big and glossy, and pure black with green eyes. Perhaps she had a touch of Burmese. We chose the biggest male, slightly long-haired, with a wide, humorous face. Then I saw Aidan eyeing the prettiest of the females, a slim, short-haired kitten that moved with unusual grace, and took fearless leaps from Phyllis's lap to the floor. Aidan was the one who said it: 'Why don't we have two? They will be company for each other.'

So now our household was complete. The cats turned out to be a very good addition. They leant a sculptural beauty to the garden, where they posed together, usually with their backs to the house. They were very easy to live with, being almost totally silent, and never cried for food. If they wanted to be fed, they sat and stared at their empty food bowls. At first they were so small they had to be carried up and down the stairs. Aidan often obliged. The young female liked to sleep on his slippered foot, leaving him, as he pointed out, like St Kevin with the blackbird, unable to move for hours. They were quickly house-trained, and once they were big enough, a friend installed a cat door so that they could come and go independently.

The tom, which had been named Mossie, a local diminutive of Thomas, turned out to be female, but we kept the name. The beauty was named Molly for the meanwhile, until we found the right name. This turned out to be Naseby, chosen by Aidan, who came across it as the name of a yellow dog in one of the Patrick O'Brian novels. Naseby was an unusually intuitive cat, and her company was often an invaluable consolation to Aidan. She persisted in her love of heights, and especially seemed to enjoy making me anxious, by climbing to dizzying heights in our apple trees or perching precariously eight feet high on our extra-tall garden pergola. Aidan decided that Chloe, the mother cat, had most likely had a tryst with an otter, and the extraordinary, fearless Naseby was the result. The silent black cats were the final piece of the jigsaw that made 2 Higher Street into a home.

★

In October 1995 it was announced that Seamus Heaney had won the Nobel Prize for Literature. I had learnt since meeting Aidan that when Seamus could not attend whatever occasion he had been invited to by a friend, he had the endearing habit of sending a postcard to apologise, and wish his friend well. Aidan had several of these. When Aidan heard about the Nobel he was delighted for Seamus, and immediately started sketching out replies in his notebook:

A tootle on the flute for Seamus Heaney, oracle of ordinary miracles and our living past. No better man to follow in the footsteps of Shaw, Yeats, Beckett onto Parnassus.
P a c h a n g a !
Salutations from Aidan Higgins and Alannah Hopkin, and all best wishes for the future.

★

Aidan's friend the artist Philomena Rafferty died in 1996 after a short illness. Aidan heard the sad news from a friend in Belfast, but too late to attend the funeral. They had been friends since 1952, when he first arrived in London. He sent a letter of condolence to her sister Agnes. Shortly afterwards there was a phone call from Agnes. She wanted Aidan's advice on what to do with all the work that Philomena had left in her studio. Aidan advised her to contact John de Vere, one of Dublin's leading fine art auctioneers, mention the Gerard Dillon connection, and invite him to come and look at the work with a view to a sale. He tracked down the address and phone number, and sent it to her.

I noticed an advertisment for her studio sale on Saturday, 15 March 1997. There were no reserves on any of the paintings, as Philomena had never exhibited in her lifetime, and was totally unknown to the public, but the auctioneer's catalogue gave estimates. Aidan thought it mean of Agnes not to have offered him a small painting in view of his long friendship with Phil, and in thanks for his help, nor even to have let him know about the sale. He went up to Dublin for the viewing, and left a bid of £250, in line with the advised estimate, on the picture of washing blowing on the line that he had liked in Omagh. When he rang on the Monday he was told it had sold for £3,800.

The sale of 160 works totalled £140,000, and according to John de Vere, almost all the pictures were bought by private buyers. Her Art Deco-inspired style had a freshness and her drawing a liveliness not unlike that of her teacher, Gerard Dillon, and appealed greatly to the art-buying public of the time. The sale was a forerunner of the great boom in contemporary Irish art of the early twentieth century.

*

Geoff Mulligan had suggested that a new edition of Aidan's short stories should be published by Minerva, Secker & Warburg's paperback imprint, under the title *Flotsam and Jetsam*. This appeared in 1997. Aidan was seldom pleased with book covers, but he very much liked this one. Its background consisted of a detail from a black and white photograph by Inge Morath of a dancer's lower legs in black shoes beneath a swirling skirt. Superimposed were the words from a review by Nuala Ní Dhomhnaill, 'The best English language prose stylist in the country.'

Flotsam and Jetsam was in fact a compromise, as there had been no paperback version of *Helsingør Station & Other Departures* or *Ronda Gorge & Other Precipices*. *Flotsam and Jetsam* included all the stories from his first book, *Felo de Se* (some under new titles), plus the new ones from *Helsingør Station*, together with an extract from *Balcony of Europe*, three repurposed travel pieces from *Ronda Gorge*, an extract from the radio play 'Texts for the Air' and a riff on Dean Swift and Esther 'Vanessa' Vanhomrigh that made use of some of the real Vanessa's letters. It might seem that this was a catchall collection, but the Irish academic Gerry Dukes, reviewing it for the *Irish Times*, enumerates the changes to the stories since first publication, and makes the perceptive point that every change that Aidan made for this new collection is turning the story away from fiction towards autobiography. And, indeed, this is the direction in which his new writing had been tending since the late 1980s.

C. L. Dallat's review in the *TLS*, while not uncritical, has a final paragraph recognising that the collection confirms Aidan's stature as a writer: '*Flotsam and Jetsam* offers a vivid illustration of Higgins's range and eclecticism, his outstanding control of atmosphere, his literary development and his importance in the history of twentieth-century Irish literature, in which he can be seen as a missing link between the modernist period and contemporary writing.'[29]

★

The wedding of Dermot Healy and Helen Gillard was to be held at the Sligo Registry Office in the Markievicz Building, a modern one, at 4.30 p.m. on Wednesday, 3 September 1997. I was surprised to find that Dermot had made elaborate arrangements, and talked with great excitement about his 'wedding car', which had been decked out in the Cavan colours for him by 'the crowd in Austies', the pub in Rosses Point, where he had been based for a while. He had invited well over a hundred and twenty people, far more than could be accommodated in the Registry Office, so there would be another gathering and more readings at the chapel on the Lissadell Estate, out near his home at Maugherow, presided over by the Reverend Gallagher, the Church of Ireland rector, and Father Kilduff from Cavan, who had been a great friend of Dermot's mother.

Many of the wedding guests spent the morning in Sligo town, and we kept running into each other. I took Aidan to the hairdresser, and went off to make some work phone calls. When I came back, Dermot was in the next seat, accompanied by a group of male supporters. We went for a drink in Hargadon's, and ran into Bill Swainson and Seán Golden. We had lunch with Bill at a road house beyond Drumcliff, then went back to our respective B&Bs, all booked for us by Dermot, to change.

The registry office was packed, and we were surprised when several people pointed Roddy Doyle out to us. He was then at the height of his fame, having won the Booker Prize in 1993 for *Paddy Clarke Ha Ha Ha*. The films of the first two novels of his Barrytown Trilogy – *The Commitments* (1991) and *The Snapper* (1993) – were hugely popular. He was the one contemporary writer that everyone in Ireland had heard of, but neither Aidan nor I had known he was a friend of Dermot's.

Roddy Doyle's success was a great mystery to Aidan. He honestly could not understand why people would want to read books that to him read like TV soap opera scripts. It didn't help that they had the same publisher, Secker & Warburg. I could see that he was both taken aback and puzzled to find Secker's star turn at the wedding.

Aidan had been asked to read 'The Snow Man' by Wallace Stevens. The final poem before the ceremony was Byron's, 'So We'll Go No More A-roving', which caused loud laughter among the company, and prompted the female registrar to remind Helen that she could still change her mind.

After more readings in the chapel at Lissadell, which was packed with guests and well-wishers, we all gathered outside Lissadell Parish Hall, where last-minute preparations of a seafood buffet from Laura's pub in Carney were still going on. Dermot had tried to get into the hall for some reason, and had been sternly told, 'You can't come in here, this is a wedding kitchen,' and was delighted to point out that he was the groom. He showed me his 'wedding car', an Austin Wolsey, with great pride. I was surprised that he had taken so much trouble with his wedding arrangements, but perhaps there was a conventional side to Dermot that I didn't really know. I was very glad that he was marrying Helen; she seemed exactly the kind of well-grounded counterbalance that he needed for the long haul, and she was also very funny. I believed they would be very happy together.

We ran into old friends, including Tony Cronin, Anne Haverty, and the novelist and poet Leland Bardwell, a great admirer of Aidan's work, who lived nearby. There was a band put together by a friend of Dermot's, and Aidan and I had two dances in the festive atmosphere, one of the few times we ever danced together, before getting into an intense conversation with the artist Seán McSweeney, another neighbour. It was not a late night, as Helen and Dermot had to travel to Dublin for an early flight to Ottawa the next morning, for a literary festival and then their honeymoon. We were meant to join everyone for a last drink at Ellen's, Dermot's local, but we couldn't find it in the maze of small back roads, and ended up at Laura's in Carney. The guards chose that night to raid Ellen's, and all the men found on the premises gave their name as 'Roddy Doyle'.

★

I had known long before the trip to New York in 1994 that Aidan was not an easy person to travel with, and from quite early days in our relationship it had to be a really tempting destination for me to agree to go with him when he was invited to read somewhere. I travelled quite a lot for my own work, and I also enjoyed being at home alone while Aidan was away. So while I was happy, for example, to have two nights in Paris when he read at the Pompidou Centre in May 1996, and to drive him to Bantry on the famous occasion when he left at home the all-important paper on which he had laboured for six weeks and was about to read, I passed on Derry, Swansea, Cheltenham and the likes. So I was not there the night that Aidan and Dermot had a major falling out late at night in October 1997 during the Cheltenham Literary Festival. When I met him at the airport on Monday evening he complained of Dermot's 'intolerable' behaviour the night before, some boisterous rough-housing involving a sheepskin jacket that alarmed a Spanish woman who thought he'd gone quite mad. Even though Dermot had apologised the next morning, Aidan was thoroughly fed up with his disruptive ways.

Nevertheless, he was in London alone once again two years later for the screening of *I Could Read the Sky*, a film by Nichola Bruce based on the novel by Tim O'Grady and Steve Pyke in which Dermot Healy stars as an old man, an Irish labourer long based in London, recalling his past. Bill Swainson, Dermot's editor, who was also there, remembers Aidan being at the Jurys hotel after-hours session following the screening. He recalls: 'Aidan went to bed angry with Dermot's drunkenness that time too, though it has to be said that Dermot was under considerable stress – he had gone into character for the film and used some aspects of that part for the main character in his novel *Sudden Times* (1999), which was launched soon after. It was as if he were caught in some shamanistic space between the two.'

So we didn't see Dermot and Helen again for quite a long time. I remember calling into Maugherow and staying the night on my own, and having a very pleasant time, but unfortunately there was a long gap before the four of us met again.

*

Our own wedding followed later that year on 20 November. For some time now we had been intending to do something about the fact that although we shared the mortgage repayments equally, the house was still in my name alone. I had of course bequeathed it to Aidan, but that would give rise to complications with tax. We went to see our solicitor, and it became apparent that the easiest way to solve the problem would be for us to get married. Neither of us objected, in fact we both liked the idea, as long as it could be done quietly in a registry office. For all the ups and downs, and there were many, Aidan made me feel loved, wanted.

I believe he felt the same; we did not discuss it because we were close enough for each to know how the other felt.

For some reason Aidan was familiar with the Cork Registry Office, a modern annexe tucked away behind a large church in a dingy corner of Cork, and declared that we could not possibly get married there. We would have to do it in Dublin. That could be arranged, provided one of us spent some time officially resident there, before the big day. Aidan volunteered for that, as I had work commitments in Cork. So we set a date about six weeks ahead. His old friends John and Nuala Mulcahy, former publishers of *Hibernia* magazine, who were delighted at the news, offered to put him up in their house while he fulfilled his residency condition. Denis, my brother and his wife Jenny, anxious to have a family presence at the 'big day', arranged to come over. Derek volunteered to be best man, as was only right and proper, having introduced us in the first place. Nuala Mulcahy was to be a witness, and Aidan decided to invite Anthony Cronin, his oldest friend. He came with his partner Anne Haverty. The Dublin registry office was on the ground floor of a Georgian town house two doors down from Buswells Hotel; as it happened, the office was closing the Friday after our wedding, and moving to a new, modern building. Quite by accident, we got our date only in the nick of time. I decided to invite our guests to champagne in Buswells, and Denis insisted on taking the remaining guests out to dinner afterwards. It was all set.

Mary Elsom, my father's youngest sister, died shortly after we'd made our arrangements. I spoke to her sons, with whom I had always been close, and assured them I would be at the funeral. I told Aidan that I would not expect him to come, as he had only met Mary a few times. But he knew that Mary and the Elsom family meant a lot to me, and he liked her, so he said he would come too. 'After all, we're practically married.' He liked the novelty of the idea, and so did I. Then my cousins contacted me with the date of the funeral: 20 November 1997, the exact same date as our wedding. I could hardly cancel my own wedding to go to a funeral. Denis and Jenny felt it was more important to be at my wedding than at Mary's funeral, so they too made their excuses. Mary, besides giving me many books over the years, had also given me a good black hat the last time I'd seen her. I decided to wear the hat to the wedding in her honour, with a black fake fur coat I had bought specially, and a long-sleeved white silk shirt I already owned.

The registrar's room was just big enough to hold our wedding party. Derek had brought buttonhole carnations for the men. It was unexpectedly touching, repeating the vows, Aidan putting on the ring, and signing the register in such a small space. We were both very happy in a quiet way: it seemed the right thing to do. We were showered with confetti afterwards, which blew everywhere as we walked the few steps up the road to Buswells Hotel in the November dusk. Luckily Jenny remembered to bring her camera. No one else, me included, had thought of making a record of the event.

The following February we spent in Mexico, at the invitation of my sister Pixie. We were royally entertained, as Aidan described so well in *The Whole Hog*. But when we were on our own, I kept things low-key and didn't press too many outings on him. Although he enjoyed the Diego Rivera murals in Mexico City and Cuernavaca, and the Museum of Anthropology, he no longer had the appetite for new discoveries. He would be seventy-one in March. New things made him edgy, ill-at-ease. We drove down to Acapulco, setting off in the dawn, on a new highway that ran through miles and miles of low hills and empty scrubland. It was a beautiful drive, with scarcely another car on the road, and rarely a peon to be seen among the hills, a sharp reminder of the sheer scale of Mexico. We were staying in a palatial house that my sister and her partner had bought as a speculative investment, just before the peso crashed, and which was currently unsaleable. They called it the white elephant, and kept it ticking over with just a house boy to mind it between holiday visits until the market picked up again. It was at La Roqueta, where Acapulco Bay reaches the open sea, and had a view of a couple of small islands. The large Art Deco-style house had long balconies designed to mimic the deck of an ocean liner. To swim, we walked down about thirty steps cut into the rock face to a wooden raft tethered on the ocean. The house boy carried a cooler full of beer and avocados down for our lunch, balanced expertly on his shoulder. We went for a siesta after lunch, and Aidan was so overwhelmed by the combination of exotic surroundings and argumentative old friends and relations that he chose not to reappear until the next day.

What he liked best in Mexico was my sister's country place near Cuernavaca, a simple ranch-style house with a carefully tended garden and swimming pool, the centrepiece of a smallholding where roses and avocados were grown. He would sit in the garden all day reading and dozing. A lunch of avocados and fresh tortillas with a couple of beers would be brought to us by the caretaker's little daughter, and as the sun went down, gin and tonic with ice and lemon would appear, followed by a simple home-cooked meal.

What I remember most about that trip was the first day I saw Aidan in shorts in the sun: his hair, which looked brown in the Irish light, was auburn, verging on red in the tropical sun. For all these years I had been living with a redhead without knowing it.

★

Already, even before he had completed *Donkey's Years*, Aidan was planning a sequel. He had found a format that suited him, the discursive autobiography, and now that he was settled with his books and old notebooks around him in his own house, he could work all the hours that he wanted.

Once again Aidan wrote *Dog Days* at a terrific pace, in less than three months. It was published in 1998, a year after we got married, and is dedicated 'For Zin, on the sunny side of the street'. Secker refused to pay for a launch, so we organised one ourselves in a pub in Kinsale, the Lord Kingsale. Aidan was by then so well known around the town that some seventy people turned out to hear him read a paper entitled 'Musing', and a short piece from the new book. A Dublin launch at the United Arts Club was organised by our friend Philip Harvey, an amiable bibliophile who had looked after Aidan's mentor Patrick Collins in his old age.

Dog Days is a sequel to *Donkey's Years* in that it contains some of the same characters, further along in life, but it is entirely *sui generis*, and like its predecessor, quite unlike any other autobiography. It opens with a kind of prelude, 'First Love', an account of the teenage Aidan's affair with an older woman, a sometime golfing partner and Montessori teacher, who refuses to allow him to consummate their passion. It is very funny, and at times quite touching. It also incorporates early memories of the Dublin of his youth. Part Two, a short section, chronicles the death of his father, soon after Aidan and his family had arrived in Berlin. Then follows a long record of the first year Aidan spent renting a cottage from a woman he calls Devorgilla, some three miles outside Wicklow town. It is based on a daily diary he kept at the time. 'The Tomb of Dreams', another short section (and also the title of one of his radio plays) is based on a diary Aidan kept in 1977, when he was back in Ireland, living on a grant from the American Irish Fund, set partly in Dublin and partly in rural Galway

One of the strengths of *Dog Days* is Aidan's acutely sharp ear for pub talk. There is an especially poignant snippet from a snug in Castlebar in a chapter called 'Halley's Comet':

> A small fierce old man with crutches by his tall stool sipped Jameson and kept watching me, at last addressed me, asking the one question to which there is no satisfactory answer: 'What do you do?'
> 'I write books actually.'
> 'What classa books?'
> 'Books that don't sell.'[30]

This was now his real-life answer to the oft-asked question, though on a really bad day he might vary it to, 'Books that nobody reads.'

Dog Days also features a comical account of Aidan's brother Colman (Colum in the book), and his wife Sylvia (Stella Veronica) in their self-built home in the Wicklow countryside. The house, designed by Colman, Senior Executive Planner of Wicklow County Council at the time, and built under his supervision, was created in accordance with his much-quoted (by Aidan) aphorism: 'Why bother about style if reality is already two-thirds illusion', a saying which I have never quite managed to fathom.

Aidan describes his first sighting of the house:

The nameless low-lying abode was on Dunganstown hill just off the narrow by-road, guarded by earthen embankments, so that you would pass and not see it from the road, for no chimney stacks were visible, no windows revealed any interior, no name (Ard ne Greine was popular all over Ireland) graced the gatepost. But it was in there all the same, crouched down and hidden by its earthworks and plantings of saplings – a cross between a Russian dacha in the woods and Robinson Crusoe's ambuscade built into a hillside, not intended to be seen.

It had the functional look of Crusoe's makeshift compound, thrown together with material that came to hand; part stockade, part granary, a homestead not drawing attention to itself, like its owner.[31]

Aidan's descriptions of the house's squalor are unflinching – rats running races above the bedroom and pissing onto the bed, 'great feculent piles of old newspapers', a slowly expiring fire that drew badly, and so on. He did not exaggerate; it really was as bad as he says. Sylvia is depicted as painfully shy, and oblivious to dirt and discomfort ('all the rooms in the house looked as if they had never been swept or cleaned'). But she does her best to welcome her long-lost brother-in-law, who reappears unannounced after a gap of ten years.

As usual, Aidan sent a copy of the new book to Colman, and was puzzled not to hear anything from him. Then came the letter. Colman was incandescent with rage: his privacy had been invaded, his wife insulted, and all of County Wicklow could read about his private life. He had gone to his solicitor, asking him to ensure that the book would be removed from all County Wicklow libraries. But his solicitor had advised that this would only give publicity to the book, and attract attention to the material that Colman was so anxious to keep quiet. So Colman had reluctantly agreed to do nothing.

Aidan was mortified; it had never occurred to him that Colman would object to having his private life written about. But now that Colman had revealed his outrage, Aidan saw his point. I blamed myself too. Because Aidan was the one writing the book, he was too close to it to be expected to foresee this reaction. I was the one who should have suggested that he run it by Colman before going to print. But because Aidan and Colman were so close, I assumed he knew Colman's limits, and was confident he would not be offended. Apparently not.

He thought it better not to phone Colman, and spent the next day writing what he called 'an abject letter of apology'. He wanted to do more, and decided to invite Colman and Sylvia to lunch somewhere midway between Wicklow and Cork, and apologise in person. A new country house hotel had just opened in Dunbrody, County Wexford, which sounded sufficiently grand for the occasion. I organised for a special vegetarian lunch to be served in a private dining room on a Saturday. We drove up in good time for the 1 p.m. appointment, but there was no sign of Colman and Sylvia. By half past two, Aidan had drunk the first bottle of white wine, with a little help from me (the driver), and ordered another. I rang Dunganstown, but there was no reply. It was almost 3 o'clock when they arrived, having, in their vague way, decided to go to an art exhibition in a nearby town that turned out to be much further away than they had thought. Or was it just vagueness? The setting and the food were highly praised by Colman and Sylvia, but there was no joy in the gathering. We drove home feeling even worse about Colman than we had done before.

The book was well received, its reception possibly even better than that given to the more conventional *Donkey's Years*. C. L. Dallat in the *TLS* judged it 'A passionate and troubling complement to Higgins's prolific output and an exemplary addition to the canon of Irish writing.'[32] It was also the book that first brought Aidan's writing to the attention of Annie Proulx, giving rise to her much-quoted review in the *Washington Post*: 'The ferocious and dazzling prose of Aidan Higgins, the pure architecture of his sentences, takes the breath out of you. He is one of our great writers. *Dog Days* is a magpie's hoard of misadventures, little grass fires of the heart and left-hand sleight. The reader who cannot take pleasure from it must be dead.' Annie Proulx is no mean hand at the dazzling prose herself.

*

On 14 June 1998 we were in Dublin for yet another Bloomsday. We went up the night before because Aidan had been invited to read at Dublin Castle with Seamus Heaney and Carol Ann Duffy, as part of the full-scale literary festival that now took place over a whole week in mid-June. How wrong the 'crypto-fascists' had been back in 1987 when they declared that the public celebration of Bloomsday would never catch on: the Bloomsday festival was getting bigger and more popular with each passing year.

We had arranged to have an early dinner that night with Derek, who was living nearby in Fitzwilliam Square. There was some confusion over the guest house booking that had been made for us by the Bloomsday Festival people, which had to be sorted out. We were going to be late leaving for the Shelbourne, where we were meeting Derek, so I told Aidan to go ahead, while I got the room organised, and changed for dinner.

On his way, Aidan ran into an old friend, Brian Mooney. He was also meeting people at the Shelbourne, so Aidan arrived in company. Derek had invited Letitia Pollard, the editor of the Irish Tourist Board's magazine, *Ireland of the Welcomes*, to join us for dinner, and had booked a table for four at La Mère Zou, a popular place nearby. Not knowing this, Aidan had suggested to Brian Mooney that he and his friends join us for dinner. By the time I arrived both Aidan and Derek were out of sorts, Aidan having had to un-invite Brian as the restaurant was unlikely to have a larger table at such short notice.

Letitia was as always full of lively conversation and news. Aidan had expected to be alone with Derek, just the three of us, like in the old days, and was not enjoying the occasion. He was also disappointed that Derek would not come to the reading the next day at Dublin Castle. Derek explained that he didn't go to other people's readings, nothing personal, he just didn't. This was not unusual among poets. Aidan suspected that the reason he would not go was because Seamus was reading, but stopped short of saying so. Instead, he started sniping at Derek, nasty little digs, until eventually I heard him say, 'I expect you were relieved to hear that the right man won the Nobel,' at which we all fell silent, shocked. Derek calmly but coldly asked, 'What do you mean by that?'

Aidan, visibly upset, had realised that he had overstepped the mark, and his comment had been taken amiss. A social gaffe, he called such mistakes. Unusually, he backtracked: 'Nothing to do with the poetry. I'm sorry. What I meant to say was that all the glad-handing that will be involved wouldn't have suited you, whereas it will come naturally to Seamus. I wasn't talking about the poetry.'

Aidan had often told Derek that he rated his work far more highly than Heaney's, so his explanation rang true. The two of them left the restaurant still friends, but it was a close thing.

PART III
'A Surly Fellow of Advanced Years'
1999–2012

2 Higher Street, Kinsale
20 August, 1998

Cher Cousin Tom,
Thanks for card and letter of July. Our place here contains no
extra bedrooms for putting up people and you must consider
that I am a surly fellow of advanced years disinclined to
cultivate new acquaintances or (least of all) distant relatives.
'Whom you would probably not enjoy taking out to dinner,'
says my dear wife.

If you wish to chance it, we go out occasionally to Casino
House overlooking Coolmaine beach, Yugoslav chef owner,
good wine list, pleasant ambience but not cheap.

Mid or late September might be the time, with tourists
departed, and B&Bs free again, should this suit yourself
and you feel up to encountering aforesaid surly party, Aidan
(or what remains of him) in the flesh.

We are great drinkers of Rioja, and plum brandy.
Meilleurs sentiments.
Rory

PS Don't believe what you may read about Kinsale being the
gourmet capital of Ireland; we have long given up eating out
here and have to look further afield. Casino has Munich lady
front of house and Yugoslav husband in kitchen.

Cousin Tom Higgins of Cartron Bay, Sligo recognises the Higgins sense of humour, and braves the 'surly fellow of advanced years', making the long trek from Sligo to Kinsale on 10 October. He is in his fifties at a guess, tall and athletic-looking, hair still brown, with a nice open face, and a lively mind. An engineer by profession, he is a lecturer in environmental studies at the Sligo Institute of Technology. He plays and coaches tennis and badminton, is also a golfer, and has written the definitive history of Irish tennis in three hefty volumes. Next he proposes to write a history of the Higgins family, which has branches in the USA and Australia, and runs to thousands. We take photos in the garden for the family album. He speaks fondly of his wife, Ursula, and their three daughters, one living in Australia. His father Syl Higgins was a first cousin of Aidan's father, Bart, and they were at Clongowes together. Aidan remembers Bart talking of cousin Syl. There is one cousin of that generation still alive, living in Longford, Teasy. She will be in touch. Cousin Tom is so nice that Aidan regrets insinuating that he should pay for the dinner, and offers to split the bill, but Tom refuses. I promise to send him the family tree of the Higgins of Springfield, which is easy enough as Aidan was the only one of the four brothers to have children – the three boys, Carl, Julien and Elwin, and now Elwin's four, the grandchildren: Paris, Yanika, Oscar and Rueben.

For many years we went for a long walk on the beach every Sunday. While Aidan would work any day of the week, or not as the mood took him, I thought it was a good idea to keep one day entirely work-free, so I never worked on a Sunday if I could help it. I liked this time to ourselves, outdoors, enjoying views of sea and sand and the birdlife. We did not settle for the nearest beach, but went to a bigger one about twenty minutes away, Coolmaine Bay, where the tide comes in for a great distance over flat sands. Depending on the time of year, the sand shifts and the beach changes shape, and there is always something new to see. Migrant birds are a feature in the winter months, large flocks of golden plovers, godwits and curlews. Sometimes people bring their horses down for a gallop, and in summer there are windsurfers.

Part of the beach-outing ritual consisted of buying our eggs from a friendly old woman called Mrs Desmond, whose farm was just before the beach. Her farm used to be a base for horse-drawn caravans back in the 1960s, and had the storm-battered remains of several holiday chalets scattered around the farmyard, and also rows of empty glasshouses. It was like a time-warp, and eerily free of people, as she had stopped taking guests many years ago. Her sons also lived on the farm, and presumably kept an eye on her, for she was very ancient. It was Mrs Desmond who told us that some new people had bought the old farmhouse across the road, and were going to open it as a restaurant. On looking more closely, I could see that vast amounts of brambles had been cleared away, the tiny cottage at its entrance painted white, and a herb garden planted.

Casino House opened in the summer of 1996, and was an immediate success. The old farmhouse had been stripped back, and decorated with great flair, in a clean-cut,

Scandinavian style. The wooden sash windows were left uncurtained, the floors were old timber or earthenware tiles, the tables had fresh linen napery and small bunches of flowers, menus were short and hand-written, while the two dining areas had different colour schemes, green or blue. The chef, Michael Relja, was Croatian, and his wife Kerrin was from Munich. When their twin daughters were born, they decided to leave Munich for a less pressured way of life. Kerrin's mother had a cottage in west Cork, exactly the kind of place they were looking for, so they decided to move to west Cork and eventually found the old farmhouse. The cooking was excellent, and not expensive by Kinsale standards. There were home-grown herbs and vegetables; garlic prawn salad was a favourite starter, or lobster risotto, followed by roast lamb, or duck served on large platters. The food and Kerrin's warm but always professional welcome, along with her considered answers to Aidan's questions about Munich, soon made it Aidan's restaurant of choice. Kerrin, quick to recognise a potentially difficult customer, made sure that his duck was always well-done, even though it annoyed her husband, the chef. She further endeared herself to Aidan by presenting him with a shot of slivovitz on the house at the end of every meal.

It was around this time, 1998, that Aidan's eyes started to give him serious trouble. When I pointed out a large flock of golden plovers flying overhead, he could see nothing. The beach, he said, was dark, whatever the weather, its features dim. Repeated eye infections were treated with drops and ointment by the local GP, but were so persistent that he was referred to the private clinic of the leading eye surgeon in Cork, Aidan Murray.

'Where did you get it?' was the first thing this gentle, grey-haired man asked Aidan at the first consultation.

'From my mother, I suppose. And you?'

I had no idea what they were talking about, but they certainly did: the name Aidan. Mr Murray was also a golfer, and admitted to reading books occasionally, so they became friends. Aidan gave Mr Murray a copy of *Langrishe*, on hearing that he had heard of it, but not read it. When *Donkey's Years* appeared, he was given a copy of that too. Cataracts were diagnosed, and duly operated on. Aidan was warned that the operation might not be the instant cure that most people experienced, and it wasn't. He could see no better after than before. And with the cataracts gone, Aidan Murray could see what he had feared: macular degeneration. Aidan would be able to see enough to get around, but his ability to read or do any sort of close work would not improve, and most likely would get worse. The frequent eye infections turned out to be caused by uveitis, a kind of secondary glaucoma in which the pressure of the eye shoots up, causing sudden, severe pain, which Mr Murray explained as the eye attacking itself. It came on unpredictably, at irregular intervals. The treatment was with local steroid injections into the tissues around the outside of the eye. It looked as if they were going into the iris itself, which is how Aidan described it, 'injections into the eyeball'. He was unflinchingly brave about them, and never complained.

The only fact that consoled Aidan was that uveitis was the same eye condition that had tormented James Joyce when he was writing *Finnegans Wake*. When Aidan's sight got worse, Mr Murray certified him as blind, in order that he should qualify for a disabled parking disc and other benefits. He liked to boast that he was 'registered blind'. We became regular fixtures at the hospital's Emergency Eye Clinic, under instructions from Mr Murray to check in there whenever uveitis flared up, and ask them to contact him. He could not have been kinder, somehow making time to see Aidan during an already busy workday. But it often involved long waits. Aidan knew all the nurses by name, and their recent histories. He talked to the other people in the queue and sympathised with their troubles. I sat and read; the quiet times in the Emergency Eye Clinic were very useful for catching up with my reviewing.

Gradually we stopped going to the beach at Sunday lunchtime. When I asked Aidan why, he explained that it was not the same any more, once he couldn't see the birds, nor the shore on the far side of the marram grass. Going to the beach only reminded him of how much his eyesight had deteriorated, so eventually we stopped altogether.

Colman's reaction to *Dog Days* was very much on Aidan's mind as he started work on what he declared to be the third and final volume of his memoirs. In an exercise that seemed to me penitential, he painstakingly typed out at least twelve pages of single-spaced letters from brother Colman. While I was gardening I used to watch him at work through the patio door of our sitting room. He sat always at the same angle, leaning slightly forward, head over typewriter, hands poised above the keys, immobile between extended bouts of typing, and he could stay there, apparently motionless, hour after hour. He had learnt to touch-type soon after leaving school, at the time that he was working in an advertising agency in Grafton Street, and could get up an impressive speed. Sometimes I crept silently into the galley kitchen behind him and made myself a snack, taking it downstairs to my desk to eat. Sometimes, usually at his suggestion, we ate together at our small, solid elm dining table. We had bought that handmade piece of furniture and his desk from a second-hand army surplus dealer; his desk was a vast table, about eight foot by three, that had come from an Irish Army officers' mess. Under it he stored cardboard boxes full of files and notebooks. I had given him my upholstered desk chair when I upgraded to a smaller model. Once he bought that table, he lost interest in improving the house, treating it as merely a machine for living in. Colman would have approved.

Aidan sent the typescript of *The Whole Hog*, the third volume of his trilogy, to Geoff Mulligan shortly before we left for Christmas in Spain. On receiving it Geoff had phoned Aidan with one important question: 'How much of this is recycled from other Higgins publications?' Geoff immediately said that the Colman letters had to go. Even so, the resulting book is 400 pages long. Once again, early memories of Springfield are trawled ('The Genesis of *Langrishe, Go Down*'), and described with comic brio. His early days in 'light industry' in west London are revisited, the old loves in Nerja, Berlin and Copenhagen revisited, South Africa and the Sharpeville Massacre, and the final end of the Anders-Higgins marriage. The Battle of Kinsale is revisited, this time as a rugby match. I understand now why Geoff asked that question. But there is also much material that appears for the first time – 'Down Mexico Way', an account of our 1998 visit to my sister, is in its idiosyncratic way a *tour de force* in the genre of memoir. He plundered the piece I had written for him in 1987 about living in Mexico City for a touching cameo picture of the younger Zin with her first husband. The final section, 'How the Century Ends', features Aidan's description of his day-to-day life in Kinsale, his daily rounds which now include increasingly frequent hospital appointments, and the physical decline of several of our older friends.

As the book progresses, its author is more and more preoccupied by thoughts of death and decay and suicide. Dead friends are listed, followed by the cause: 'Harry Calnek, my old amigo, did away with himself at Malaspina Road on the Powell River in British Columbia, after alerting the local police as to his intentions and the whereabouts of his remains. He had bad cancer, which had also killed Howard Simpson.'

Death looms larger and larger as the memoir proceeds, yet the tone is sprightly and resigned, the gaze steady; there is even some grandstanding. This is the beginning of the Epilogue:

Age does us no favours. Advancing years do not bring serenity; our end is as likely to be as untidy and messy as our beginning, when we came bawling messily into this world.

The carnal clinch can be left behind as an embarrassment. Eyesight failing. Teeth gone to pot, bridges installed; hearing only so-so, memory likewise, nostrils and ears sprouting hair, pubics offer scant cover; the metabolism getting into the swing of it before the final dissolution, the final descent into the grave, to be scattered as ashes about some favoured spot, tipped into some river, lake or sea.[1]

There follows a graphic description of the fate of those who opt for the grave, which is worth persevering with for the change of tone at its conclusion:

Coffin boards are removed elsewhere by busy termites, wriggling worms going at it; human bones scattered all over the place, appendages – eyeless sockets and hairless skulls – dropping off and devoured in our final dissolution into the teeming earth. We all roll with the earth's turning, asleep forever on its broad, deeply breathing bosom. Thinking of dead friends is the price we pay for our rest.[2]

On a personal level, I like the book for his affectionate portrait of my sister in Chapter 63, 'The *Zaca* Sails Again!' This marks an important turning point, because she and Aidan had not always got on well. He found her bossy and manipulative, and resented the time I spent with her on her infrequent visits. But from here on, it was all – well almost all – sweetness and light between them.

And, of course, I like the tribute he paid to me, as the last and greatest of his *amours*. He did not write about me much, for the simple reason that once we met, I was always there. 'Zin is in,' as he liked to say, when I came back from one of my sorties. His other 'loves' were mostly remarkable for their absence, his love a matter of longing and dreams.

*

In September 1999 we went to Nerja again. I was about to turn fifty, and much as I liked my friends, I didn't want to have the round of celebrations that would be expected if I stayed in Kinsale. The landmark birthday seemed to have arrived too soon. I surely wasn't old enough to be fifty?

Paulette was now a widow. Donal, on being diagnosed with terminal cancer, had decided to kill himself, to save Paulette the trauma of nursing him, a task that she proclaimed she would have been well up to. He accumulated enough pills, and took them with an amount of fine brandy while they were at Paulette's family home, Saint Amour. Paulette did not go to Nerja the following summer, but she kindly offered us the use of her apartment, 'to celebrate the birthday of George Sand'.

My brother Denis and Jenny were staying near Marbella, and came over for the big day. Denis invited us out to dinner at the Parador, which was only a short walk away, above Burriana beach. In return, we were able to offer them a bed for the night. Once again, Jenny was the only one with a camera, and we are pictured at the end of the meal behind a formidable display of empty glasses, having started with an aperitif of *manzanilla*, and sampled several wines before reaching the cognac stage – for those who indulged. I had realised that I was better off without spirits in my life, and had not drunk any for seven or eight years. I had also stopped smoking, largely because Aidan had predicted that I would never kick the habit.

When we were alone in the apartment we lived much as we did at home, Aidan going off in the morning to the Balcony of Europe, an elegant marble-tiled walkway jutting out into the sea, dating from Napoleonic times, for his coffee and cognac, while I read in the sun, then swam. Sometimes we'd go for a walk in the late afternoon: he showed me several places that featured in *Balcony of Europe* – La Luna, a bar-café in the 1960s, which was now an expensive restaurant on the edge of town, and the old town cemetery, with its dovecote-like slots for ashes. One afternoon we walked, as did Ruttle and Charlotte, from Burriana to Maro, a distance of about five kilometres. The sun was unusually hot and Aidan was now having trouble with high blood pressure, and any unusual exertion left him dizzy and tired for the next day or two. He was no longer keen on sea swimming, preferring the security of the apartments' communal pool.

In the evenings we listened to Donal's music collection, mainly classical, on his excellent sound system, and read or dozed. Sometimes we went out around 10 p.m. to observe the street life, mostly quiet couples sharing a drink. One time we had our photographs taken on the main square with our heads through the holes of a wooden flat of a couple dressed as flamenco dancers, which greatly amused us both.

Some old friends from Kinsale, Jill and Don Herlihy, had a holiday home in Nerja in a small development quite near our building, called Miramar. Jill had told me that her next-door neighbour, a German woman, on hearing that she lived in Ireland, had asked if she knew an Irish writer called Aidan Higgins. 'Of course,' said Jill. 'He's married to my friend Alannah.'

I had given her our phone number at Paulette's, so Jill invited us over for drinks, and naturally she asked her German neighbour who knew Aidan Higgins, and her husband, to join us. So it was that one evening soon after my birthday I found myself having poolside drinks with Jill and Don, Aidan's former lover, Hannelore, and her husband, Klaus Boykens. Aidan had worked out that the Hannelore Boykens mentioned by Jill Herlihy must be his ex from Berlin in 1966. So he knew what to expect, though he had never warned me. But that was typical: in the same way, he had never clearly explained where we were going, the day that he took me to visit Springfield.

Hannelore features as Hanne or Lore in the stories, and in *Lions of the Grunewald* she is the woman for whom Aidan left his wife and three small children while living in Berlin. She was his second great obsession after Charlotte/Harriet of *Balcony of Europe* (or third, if you count Jill/Nancy, his wife), and here she was in Nerja, in the wrong novel, so to speak. The huge scale of the coincidence had not yet sunk in while we sat by the pool with our Kinsale friends, sipping our drinks, and I was (naïvely) surprised that Aidan took it so calmly.

Klaus and Hannelore were typical of the kind of wealthy, low-key north Europeans who are attracted by a quiet resort like Nerja, which lacks both the ostentation of Marbella, and the mass tourism that has ruined much of the coast between there and Málaga. She seemed, perhaps, older than him, tall and skinny, x-ray like, pale and blonde, dressed in white, with long white hair, worn loose with a 1960s' fringe. She could have been the ghost of Hannelore. Klaus was dark-haired and sallow with a receding hairline, medium-height like Aidan, not overweight, but sleek and well-fed in comparison to his wife. He was a medical consultant, and worked in Berlin for six months of the year. The rest of the time they divided between Cuba, where he volunteered his medical expertise, and Nerja, where they both relaxed. 'Hannelore cannot take the cold anymore,' he explained, in his perfect English.

We arranged to meet again, for dinner this time, at Klaus's preferred restaurant, a quiet neighbourhood place that we had already discovered. I had still not quite grasped the fact that I was dining with the famous Hannelore. I neither liked nor disliked her, having hardly spoken to her, but it didn't matter. I knew what was going to happen at the dinner: Aidan would monopolise his old love, Hannelore, and I would be left to talk to Klaus. Hannelore had barely acknowledged my existence. Luckily, I liked Klaus, and we had plenty in common. He had a wide knowledge of the symphony orchestras, conductors, concert halls and opera houses of Europe, and he also had first-hand knowledge of Cuban life after the revolution, especially its excellent health system.

When the bill arrived, Klaus picked it up. When Aidan protested and offered to share it, he was waved away. Aidan resumed his conversation with Hannelore, while Klaus explained with a wry expression: 'Do not think this is the first time I have taken an ex-boyfriend of Hannelore's out to dinner. I am well used to it. And I always pick up the bill. She had a knack for knowing men who never made any money. Until she met me!' Klaus looked very pleased with himself, and I liked him for smirking as he made this strange admission.

★

We were in Nerja again for Christmas 2000. We had decided to shorten the Irish winter by spending six weeks in Spain, starting in early December. A couple of Americans we had met, who were living in Kinsale on their yacht, would be happy to move into our house and look after the cats.

By asking around in Nerja, I found Paco, a caretaker, who could rent us a fifth-floor apartment a short walk from Paulette's, with a balcony and a great view over the sea and the nearby hills. The décor was dowdy and old-fashioned, early 1960s perhaps, but the rent, cash in hand, was extremely reasonable, and it was clean and well-equipped. When Paulette came over to take a look, she pointed to the volumes of Maigret on the bookshelves. 'Belgian,' she said, 'the owners are Belgian, and of a certain age, perhaps too old to come here anymore. Many Belgians invested in Nerja in the early days. And Canadians. Now they leave the keys with a caretaker like Paco, he sublets, and sends them some money from time to time, and everybody is happy.'

'*Todos contentos y yo tambien,*' I said. George Sand was helping Paulette to improve her Spanish.

Aidan's ex-wife Jill, who had a house in the hills above Nerja, and his middle son, Julien, who lived in Valladolid, were coming to stay with Paulette for Christmas, and we would all spend it together. It worked well. Jill and I kept our distance; there was no warmth, but neither was there any hostility. Aidan always enjoyed seeing Julien, and since Julien had moved in with Marisa in Valladolid, Aidan seemed to have stopped worrying about his future.

There had been another suicide since Aidan and Jill had last met: Harry Calnek, a newspaperman and writer, one of Aidan's walking *compañeros* from Nerja in the late 1960s. I never met him, but he sounds like a gentle soul with a lively sense of humour, and a wry turn of phrase. His sad end is described in *The Whole Hog*. He had asked for his ashes to be scattered near Cómpeta, the village in the hills above Nerja, where many people, including Jill, had retreated as the coast became too expensive. Donal, one of his oldest friends, was now referred to by Aidan as 'Donal the suicide', while Harry's name was seldom mentioned without the additional information, 'he shot himself with a point two-two in British Columbia'.

Christmas at Paulette's went well. Between us we cooked a small turkey with chestnut stuffing and no other trimmings. Julien, a quiet, dreamy man in his late thirties, was a teacher of Spanish and of English, who wanted to write. He had tried stories, and was now writing short poems. He had inherited Aidan's eternal youthfulness, and looked about twenty-five. He had seen very little of Aidan since he had moved to Kinsale, and I was glad they could spend time together. He organised the order of ceremony on Christmas Day, including the distribution of presents, with childlike enthusiasm. His partner Marisa (who was not with us) had introduced him to the Spanish art of present-giving, and their offerings were carefully chosen.

It rained heavily on Christmas Eve, followed by a storm of thunder and lightning. Aidan was unsettled in our Belgian apartment. Although it was only a six-minute walk from Paulette's apartment – familiar territory – he could not find his way home alone. Knowing this, he had written down the name of our building, Edificio Capri, and our street, Bella Vista, and kept the note with his keys. The balcony, which had at first delighted him, was now a source of terror, and its railing had to be draped with a beach towel to disguise the height before he could be tempted out. He had a new dental plate, and could be heard in the bathroom, gagging and choking, morning and evening, as he tried to master putting it in and taking it out. He said nothing to me, beyond reporting his inability to find his way home, but I could see that he was in a state of high anxiety. When I read his diary (in 2019 in the Harry Ransom Center in Austin, Texas) I found this note:

> Too fearful to look over balcony five storeys up. Down and down, the compass needle dead on terror. Can hardly open a door, order coffee, calculate the correct tip, find the way home. Helpless. A vacancy of spirit, a terror of the unknown, the foreign here and now whose language you cannot speak. The tower of San Isidro church, bell rings as punishment, a flogging. Wakefulness and sleeping, anxieties crowd in, overpower me.

I had no idea of the extent of his suffering at that time. I just thought he was unusually nervous. I remember making a big joke about his deteriorating Spanish when he ordered 'Dos coffees, por favor,' not suspecting that he was in such a fragile state.

That Christmas, as usual, I bought two page-a-day diaries, one each, for 2001. He did not write a single word in his, and never kept a diary again. He was seventy-three, but all of a sudden, he seemed much older.

Talking in Bed
It is just before dawn in Higher Street on an early spring day. Aidan has been getting up early to witness the dawn in our garden. It is still dark and very cold. He presses me to get up with him, and go out to welcome the dawn. I tell him it is too early for me, and too cold, and turn over to go back to sleep. He says as if talking to himself, but knowing very well that I can hear him: 'Wouldn't it be a terrible thing if I had married a dull woman and didn't know it?'

I am meant to react, he is winding me up, but I will not fall into the trap. I act as if I had not heard, and turn my face into the pillow.

It was a nasty thing to say, but even so, it amuses me that he subscribes to the Dublin belief that being dull is the worst possible fault anyone can have. To me the worst fault someone can have is to be unkind. Wouldn't it be a terrible thing if I had married an unkind man and didn't know it?

Alannah's Diary, 1 March 2001
Aidan has been taken off beta-blockers after twelve years, and is having very strange reactions. We went to a concert by the Vanbrugh Quartet on the UCC campus. He is on edge, but is interested by the first half, Shostakovich's String Quartet No. 3. In the interval we walk in the quadrangle, as there are several people at the concert whom I know, including the editor of UCC's staff magazine, whom I work for regularly, and he does not want to

have to make small talk. We take different seats for the second half, a late Beethoven quartet, further back. He cannot settle, keeps shuffling in his seat, puts his head in his hands, raises his eyes to heaven and imitates a sawing, fiddle-playing motion in the air with both hands: it is going on too long for him, going on and on forever. He starts to mutter, and soon he will be talking aloud, disturbing the musicians. I wait tensely for the break after the first movement, and hustle him out of the door. Outside, he raises his arms to the sky and says, 'Thank God! I thought they were never going to stop sawing away ....'

I lost my temper completely and roared at him, 'Don't you ever do that to me again, ever!' I was about to grab his hands to make sure he was listening to me, when I was grasped firmly by the upper arms by two security guards, one on each side, asking me to come along quietly, there was a concert going on in there. 'It's him, not me, he's the problem, I had to take him out because he was going to make a scene, it's not *my* fault.' They really didn't care, as long as I left the campus without causing any more trouble. On the way home, Aidan encouraged me to drive faster, 'Wouldn't that be a nice way to go, go on, put your foot down, don't be a coward!' Then he tried to open his door and throw himself out, 'Come on, come with me, this is my idea of fun, not that interminable sawing ....' Alarmed by his behaviour, I had automatically locked all the doors before we set off. When we got home I told him, 'I am never, ever going to a concert with you again. Never.'

*

Although he had never been religious, Aidan had taken to praising God for the beauty of the days, and wishing that he still had his faith, so that he could pray. One especially fine spring day, he asked me to do him a favour, come out to the garden and throw a bucket of cold water over his head. The beauty of everything was too much for him, and he wanted to be taken back down to reality. I obliged, and he thanked me. That evening when he had gone to bed – earlier than me, because he was getting up so much earlier – I rang my sister-in-law, Jenny, who is a GP, and described his behaviour. At first she found it funny, then she said, more seriously, that it sounded as if he was suffering from some kind of mania, and I should take him to the GP, who would investigate. Meanwhile, I should encourage him to keep regular hours if possible, and lead a quiet life. No parties, no unusual outings. A quiet routine, moderation in all things, especially alcohol, and meals at regular intervals.

I made an appointment with David, our GP. Aidan objected to being taken to the doctor because he was happy. He found the absurdity of it funny, and went on and on about it. When I was tired of listening to him, he phoned several friends to tell them about this strange world, where happy people are sent to see the doctor because there must be something wrong with them. Our GP David, recognising some form of mania beyond his competency to treat, referred Aidan to a consultant psychiatrist, Dr Mairead. She couldn't see us for a couple of weeks, but asked me to keep a list of symptoms meanwhile. Here it is:

> *Time stretching and shrinking*
> *Euphoria alternating with rage and frustration*
> *Hypersensitivty to domestic noise, e.g. cupboard doors closing, chairs scraping*

Total self-absorption
Lack of concentration
Feast or famine: all high drama, every meal either the greatest
ever or the worst
Glittery eyes, new endearments that quickly turn sarcastic,
e.g. Sweetie Pie
Knuckle-biting, sobbing, lack of inhibitions
Total lack of interest in anything but himself

Dr Mairead saw us together initially in her plush rooms in
Bishopstown, a prosperous Cork suburb. Then she talked to
me on my own, and then to Aidan alone. Neither of us was
very impressed by her on that first visit. I suspected that she
found me an unreliable witness, exaggerating his behaviour,
and I suspected that Aidan was going to run rings around
her, she seemed so trusting and guileless. She ordered a
brain scan, and put him on medication. The medication
helped, and by May he was slowly coming back to his usual
self. The mania was revealed as a grotesque exaggeration
of his usual self; the short distance between the two was
frightening.

Alannah's Diary, Summer 2001
I am finding all this drama very difficult to live
with. The disorder that comes with *la locura* (I am
reluctant to use the word madness) is reflected in
the disorder of the house, normally so tidy, and
the disorder of our regime. I have never lived with
anyone who is not fully sane before, and I find it
alarming. I am living on my nerve ends too. I never
know if he will be up at crack of dawn or sleep
in until midday. I have started to drink wine after
supper as well as with the meal, staying up as late

as he does in the hope of keeping him grounded. Last night he drank almost half a bottle of brandy after supper, and oddly enough had no hangover this morning. He said he felt great, apart from the dehydration.

Chaos is a pit which has a right side and a wrong side. So far we are on the right side, where you can survive, but for how long?

With sedation comes a loss of acuity, a loss of short-term memory and a tendency to confusion – which has been there for a while – getting lost in Nerja, for example. He looks cross and exasperated at my stupidity when I don't hear what he has just mumbled. He has a tendency to disappear into another, vividly imagined world. I hate leaving him alone, even for a day, but what a relief it is too, not to be constantly monitoring his moods.

An artist friend who is training to be a Lacanian psychotherapist says, 'You do realise, he's not going to get better? He'll always be psychotic from now on; it's his age.' She completely fails to realise what a devastating thing she's just said, when I was still optimistic that he would return to normal.

How beautiful the countryside is at this time of year. May blossom, new green leaves on the beech tree translucent in the sunshine, and how alienated I feel from it. I wonder how all this natural beauty can persist, and he not be right?

At the follow-up appointment, Dr Mairead, having studied the brain scan, talks of brain shrinkage, loss of grey matter due to alcohol consumption over the years, which could account for the increasingly frequent instances of memory loss (he couldn't remember Derek's name, nor the title of *Bornholm Night-Ferry*), and the occasional confusion. Alcohol suppresses serotonin, she says, which is why it is not advisable to drink heavily in a depression, which she seems to think is inevitably going to follow the elation. When I was alone with her, she said she finds him less stormy this time, less tense, less hypomanic, though she can't use that term to him, and I agree. She starts to show some sense of humour, always useful when dealing with Aidan. She is less wary of him this time, less shy. She seems to trust me more too. When we are alone she explains that the brain scan shows underlying arterial disease, hardening of the arteries, the beginnings of a dementia-type disease – progressive, but stop-start. Relative to the state of the damage shown by the brain scan, he is doing very well. It is not Alzheimer's disease, which is all downhill, leading to total loss of personality. He will have bad times, with better times in between. The dementia could be a long time developing. There is no medication for early memory loss, but he can see a geriatrician for long-term care. The odd changes in mood probably have a physical origin, rather than originating in psychosis.

I find I am much more reconciled to the long haul with this knowledge, and no longer panic at the prospect. It helps that already he is much more the man I know, much closer to the old Aidan. But he doesn't like me to refer to him as Aidan these days, as I do sometimes when tallking to other people. 'Aidan? Who is that?' As he did at dinner with Howard and Mary Alice, he insists that we all call him Rory.

It is odd how the cats know he is not right. They sit in unusual places, look at him warily, scurry in and out by strange routes. Naseby, his familiar, is especially susceptible.

By October he is well enough to start work again, and decides to type up some old notebooks he has found, to get back into the habit of work. I remind him that today is the day, and he says, 'Brendan Behan once told me there's a woman in Wellington Road who'll give you a room for free if she hears the typewriter going. So what I do is I type a chapter of *The Brothers Karamazov* every week, and it pays the rent.'

From my room downstairs once again I hear the familiar sound of Aidan upstairs going tappety-tap, tappety-tap, the steady rhythm indicating good progress.

Everything is going to be alright.

★

The Whole Hog was published in autumn 2000, and was warmly received. It was a substantantial book of 400 pages, and once again Aidan approved of the dust jacket. It featured an atmospheric photograph by Marc Atkins of the rear view, off-centre, of a woman in a two-piece swimsuit, dreamily paddling in the blue sea under a blue sky.

Most reviewers found a few bones to pick with Rory of the Hills, disliking his return to familiar territory (childhood, the genesis of *Langrishe*, Rory amours, cranky pronouncements on the 'new Ireland', for example), while recognising the overall achievement of the three books. John Kenny in the *TLS* was typical in his summary:

Higgins has remained particularly faithful to the Joycean idea of the multiple-styled book, and here his material is richly anecdotal, epistolary, diaristic, touristic, journalistic and straightforwardly novelistic. Philosophically vagrant, learnedly jocular in the mode of Flann O'Brien or the early Beckett, he can be uproariously vulgar and vain, lavishly masculine.[3]

★

After Dr Mairead's intervention, Aidan was still on various medications, still prone to anxiety and insomnia, but in general easier to live with than when the hypomania was active. But the fading eyesight, bad hearing and poor memory had taken their toll, and I often felt he was struggling to keep up with the conversation when we saw friends, and especially when there were more than one or two people around. When a letter arrived informing him that he had been awarded an honorary DLitt by the University of Ireland, he was not as pleased as I thought he would be. It seemed to me an appropriate tribute to someone who was largely self-educated, and that he should accept. And so he did. The ceremony was held on 10 May 2001, with the campus of UCC in colourful bloom, and he was flanked by eleven good friends for the lunch that preceded the ceremony. Perhaps it would have meant more if he had invited Colman, but relations were still frosty.

Each of the nominees had to make an impromptu speech after the lunch, and he carried it off brilliantly. He looked the part in his colourful doctor's robes and velvet hat. His proposer, our friend Gerry Wrixon, recently elected President of University College Cork, spoke of him in glowing terms. Everybody clapped and congratulated him. But I suspected that he had not enjoyed a single moment of the long day. He was very relieved when it was all over. We went away together for a week, staying at a cottage on Beara belonging to Joachim and Katherine Beug. He could still read outdoors in strong sunlight, and we went for long, peaceful walks around the coast.

Aidan was surprised but pleased in September 2001 when *The Whole Hog* was shortlisted for the *Irish Times* non-fiction prize. It didn't win; the prize went to Angela Bourke for *The Burning of Bridget Cleary*, an excellent piece of work, both scholarly and readable. William Trevor's latest collection, *The Hill Bachelors*, won the Irish fiction prize. Michael Longley's *The Weather in Japan* won the poetry award, while Michael Ondaatje picked up the International Fiction Prize for *Anil's Ghost*.

Aidan was invited to Dublin to give a reading at the Irish Film Institute and attend the prize-giving, which was to be held at the Royal Dublin Society the following evening. The IFI was very busy on the night, and the arrangements fairly chaotic. We sat in the front row with William Trevor, who had come direct from the airport with a small overnight bag.

Aidan made the following announcement before his reading: 'Last December my eyesight began to deteriorate. I am afflicted with cataracts, uveitis and macular degeneration, and the wonder is that I can see at all. Reading has become very difficult and slow, and a public reading would be a fiasco. My wife has volunteered to read instead of me.' I was introduced by John Banville, who kindly referred to me as 'herself a distinguished writer and critic'. I hoped no one would complain at getting me instead of Aidan. At the end of the reading I gestured to Aidan, who deserved the applause more than me, and he came and took my hand and led me off the stage.

William Trevor read next, and asked me to hold his hat while he did so. I was amused to be sitting there minding William Trevor's well-worn pork pie hat. I wished I could keep it as a souvenir. Then there was a long wait for a taxi. There was a taxi shortage at that time; it was Friday night and raining. We were all staying in Bewley's Hotel at Ballsbridge. William and Aidan had both had a long and tiring day, and started to get grumpy as we sat on tiny chairs at a tiny corner table, waiting for the taxi.

'You may be a year older than me, but you don't have arthritis,' said William.

'No, but I'm blind as a bat,' said Aidan.

'I bet you didn't have a 5 a.m. start?'

'You have me there.'

The taxi, when it arrived, had loud music on its radio. As usual, Aidan asked politely for the music to be turned off, and it was. William always remembered this detail whenever I saw him again: he said he would never have dared to ask a Dublin taxi driver to turn off the music, but Aidan did it with such style and such conviction that no taxi driver could refuse.

The next day, because it was almost our fourth wedding anniversary, we treated ourselves to lunch at Roly's Bistro, of which we had both read good reports. Aidan was far better than I was at remembering our wedding anniversary, and arranging a celebration. We then had a meeting with our new agent, Jonathan Williams, who was keen to get Aidan's earlier work back into print. Secker had not asked for another book after *The Whole Hog*, and Aidan had nothing particular in mind. But he still had his collected criticism and his radio plays that had never been published. There had been interest in reprinting his work for the American market from John O'Brien of the Dalkey Archive Press, which Jonathan said would be a very good move. Jonathan had also taken on a story collection that I had put together, and had some editing suggestions to talk over.

The reception at the RDS was very big and well-attended. We came across many old friends, including Robin Robertson, Michael Longley and, of course, Caroline Walsh, the *Irish Times'* literary editor. I saw Eileen Battersby in the distance, but didn't get a chance to talk to her. Aidan was seated at Caroline's table, and complained afterwards that it was full of women talking about their gynaecological problems. Seated between Caroline's husband, the novelist James Ryan, and the Irish-language poet Cathal Ó Searcaigh I had no lack of lively talk. Caroline told me years later that she had been terrified all evening that Aidan might discover Eileen's presence, and take up the question of the *Helsingør Station* review again. Still, even twenty years later, he occasionally sent a sarcastic letter to the 'humourless feminist' who had turned the whole of Dublin against him.

*

In February 2002 we were in Fuerteventura, on a two-week break in a villa on the beach. I had kept myself going in the preceding winter by repeating the words 'villa on the beach', as I went about my weekly routine as a freelance arts journalist in dark, rainy Cork. We hired a car for a few days, and drove up to the old capital of the island, which was located in its mountainous interior, as a defence against pirate raids. We came into the pretty colonial town during a rainstorm, Gypsy Kings blasting out of the car's stereo, with all the lights blazing as I tried to locate the windscreen wipers. We were laughing in delight to discover a real, working village here, so different from the commercialised coast. We had a coffee, then went into a rough-hewn gallery, and bought four heavy handmade plates in an old traditional style, and a matching set of jug and coffee pot. It was a totally impractical thing to do, as we'd be flying home, but I went along with Aidan's suggestion because it was good to see him taking an interest in domestic matters again.

We arrived home to discover that our friend Thomas O'Leary had died. We knew he had been diagnosed with cancer, and had refused any treatment ('I shall proceed to forget what you have just told me,' he said to the GP who had given him the diagnosis), but we had not expected him to go so soon. Then a young friend of mine, Sophie Brem, died at very short notice, cancer again. Aidan hardly knew her, so he stayed at home, but I felt I should go to Sophie's funeral mass. Seeing her two small children so puzzled, and her husband trying to comfort them, was awful. As I left the church, several people asked if I was coming to the 'afters' in Crackpots, a restaurant near my house. I hadn't intended to, but it seemed like a good idea, with all the grieving, to be among her friends at the wake. So I went along, but I only stayed about half an hour. As I left, our friend Sarah Filhol said she'd come too, say hallo to Aidan, and freshen up at my place before her long drive home.

I knew the minute I opened the front door that something was wrong. It was one of those dark winter days with a persistent drizzle, and the cold and damp seemed to have got into the house. Upstairs, I saw that the patio doors from the house to the garden were wide open, and Aidan's shoes thrown down by the sofa. I could see him under the apple tree in a red sweater and his stockinged feet, his back to the house, the cat Naseby looking up at him, he looking up at the sky, and down at something in his hand. It was a large kitchen knife. His eyes were shut tight, and he was moaning, at the point of collapse. We walked him back to the house, supporting him on either side, encouraging him on when he wanted to stop.

We were just in time; he hadn't even broken his skin. I was so glad to have Sarah there; she had served in the American Foreign Service in Central America and could be relied on to stay calm in an emergency. She was a friend of the Simpsons, about my age, a face familiar from many parties, and I hoped her cheerful presence would help to bring Aidan back down to reality. I gave him a drink of water, and rang the GP practice. Meanwhile, he had decided he was going to throw himself off the balcony, and we had to restrain him, and lock the door. Doctor Katy arrived, with Valium. I rang Joachim, who came straight over, once he had understood my babbling. Several times Aidan tried to get out of the door again, and dash himself onto the concrete yard. I thought he was play-acting, but Joachim, who grappled with him, said he really meant it. The GP told me I would have to commit him, since he was unlikely to sign the forms himself in this state. I rang Colman, to distract Aidan, and give us time while the Valium took effect. Doctor Katy contacted the Gardaí, and persuaded them to drive Aidan to Cork in a squad car, even though strictly speaking it was not allowed. I sat in the back seat, Aidan wedged in the middle between me and a burly guard. We were driven to Ward GF, the psychiatric ward, which is at a slight remove from the main hospital.

The admission process was painfully slow, with many questions that I could not answer, and Aidan would not. But in time, he calmed down, and signed the voluntary admission form without a murmur. He promised to stay in as long as they wanted him to, and not to run away. He was given a plate of warm chicken and rice, a nice thought, as he had not eaten since breakfast. By 8 p.m. he was settled in a bed, and I headed home in a taxi. The driver was a moonlighting traditional musician, who talked all the way to Kinsale. I wanted to say, 'I have just left my beloved husband in the psychiatric ward, and I don't know if he'll ever be right again. I have never been more miserable in my life. Please shut up.' But I didn't. On the table I found an almost illegible note:

> *Goodbye dearest Zin, cannot face the long weary years ahead when you might tire of your ever loving Moulty.*

Aidan was in the psychiatric ward for three weeks. There is a good account of his time in there in *Blind Man's Bluff*. Three weeks is the usual length of stay, I was told. If you go in as a suicide, you are taken very seriously. Having been at Killashee (prep school) and Clongowes, Aidan was well able for the day-to-day routine. His natural curiosity about other people distracted him from his own woes, and his compassion for the sadder cases – a gentle teenager with a record of multiple suicide attempts, a young man who lived mainly under his bed and collected plastic bags – brought out the best in him. He was nicknamed 'Rip van Winkle' because he slept so much. Visits from friends were not encouraged by the psychiatric team, though Gerry Wrixon managed to spend some time with him.

Jenny, my medical sister-in-law, was optimistic, telling me, 'Once they get the medication right, he'll be good as new, like a diabetic whose insulin has to be right.' It seems the oral steroids he was given for his eyes by Mr Murray's locum were partly to blame.

I could not believe Aidan had seriously planned to kill himself by cutting his throat with a kitchen knife, sober and in broad daylight. It was a dramatic gesture, a cry for help perhaps, or just an expression of his all-round confusion. He was unhappy, anxious, disturbed, but not mad the way his fellow inmates were. The litanies of dead friends towards the end of *The Whole Hog* had perhaps unhinged him, made him feel that he should make a grand gesture towards earning himself a place on the list.

I phoned Dermot Healy in Sligo to let him know what had happened. A few days later, Dermot's wife Helen rang me: Dermot was in the psychiatric ward of Sligo General Hospital in the throes of a breakdown that sounded far more serious than Aidan's. I rang Aidan's three sons; the youngest, Elwin, who was working with troubled teenagers, was the only one who seemed to understand what I was saying, and sounded terribly dejected.

The psychiatrist in charge reported that Aidan's case was far from the standard suicidal impulse due to depression. She had observed a certain element of calculation in his demeanour, and I had also experienced what I refer to in my journal as 'craftiness' in his behaviour, such guile being absent from the normal Aidan. She was also aware of him turning on the charm. She asked me to ring his family to see if there had been any psychotic incidents in his past or that of his brothers. Jill told me of a time in Cómpeta when he had taken to howling at the full moon while trembling uncontrollably, something to do with a Danish girlfriend. And his brother Desmond had been in a residential institution for a period in his late teens with what sounded like a depression. Neither fact was much help.

The neighbours, dubbed by Aidan 'the noddies', a covey of tidy, grey-haired women, who gossiped on the street corners, were all concern: 'Was that your husband taken away by the guards, yesterday? We thought it was Kitty next door, her nerves have gone.' I explained it was a bad reaction to some steroids. They all nod: 'Ah the creature! How is he today, bless his heart.'

Aidan was home in three weeks, but still prone to dramatic highs and lows. No more Dr Mairead and the plush waiting room: his suicide attempt meant that he was discharged into the more rigorous care of the Southern Health Board's psychiatrist, and had to attend a fortnightly appointment in a local clinic. So now 'the shrink' was added to the round of medical appointments, eye, heart and head, pills and eye drops, uppers and downers, round and round and round, the waiting rooms, the hospital corridors, and, in between, calming interludes for me, wandering among the tidy racks of new clothes in the Bishopstown Dunnes Stores. I seldom bought anything, but I liked the sense of order in this quiet emporium, the way that nothing had a history, everything was new, unsullied. I treated it as a kind of 'decontamination chamber', a place to gather myself together, a neutral interlude between the tedious world of hospital corridors and waiting rooms, and the volatile and unpredictable atmosphere of home.

*

Caroline Walsh at the *Irish Times* sent me a book to review called *Light Years* by Augustus Young, a discursive autobiography about growing up in Blackrock, a Victorian riverside suburb of Cork city, in the 1950s and 1960s. I loved it, and said so. It was quoted on the cover of his next book: 'I have not laughed so much since my first reading of *The Third Policeman* ... this book is an oddity, but a beautiful oddity, which goes from high comedy to deep pathos in the flick of a semi-colon. The final impression is of a haunting sadness, as in all the best comic writing.'

In real life Augustus Young was an epidemiologist called James Hogan, working for the National Health Service, and also a very fine poet with a small but dedicated following. He had recently taken early retirement and moved with his wife, Margaret, known as M, from Hendon to Port-Vendres in south-west France, near the Spanish border. In the summer of 2002, I arranged a launch for James's book during the newly established Kinsale Arts Week. Aidan had enjoyed *Light Years* almost as much as I did, and was looking forward to meeting its author.

In a piece he wrote after his visit to Ireland, James observes that Aidan never quite finishes his books and compares him to a lion: 'The glint of brilliance cracks through thick spectacles. But there is something in his posture, though formally relaxed, that suggests he is about to spring.'

*

Peter Murray, as Director of the Crawford Municipal Gallery, was commissioning a series of portraits of Cork writers, by up-and-coming artists. He decided to commission Suzy O'Mullane, who had her first solo show six years before, to paint Aidan. I knew Suzy already as a live wire on the Cork art scene, whose work, mainly representative, with a distinctive, faux-naïf character, was clearly following its own path. Slim and edgy, always attractively turned out, with an intense engagement in whatever she is doing, Suzy came to the house to meet Aidan, and they seemed to like each other. He agreed to a total of six three-hour sittings in the studio at her house in Blackrock. But once she had left, he was not as enthusiastic as I had hoped. He was hiding it from me, but he had still not fully recovered from his stay in the psychiatric ward. He would often complain about how hard he found it to write with 'failing eyesight' and 'defective memory', and I sympathised. He didn't tell me about his private devils, and his increasing dependency on me, but he told Suzy.

For logistical reasons, the work had to be done at Suzy's house, which was not easy to reach by public transport. So I drove Aidan over, and wrote notes downstairs at the kitchen table, while he and Suzy worked in the third-floor attic. I was getting started on a new piece of fiction, either a long story or a short novel, and it was useful to be away from my usual surroundings, with a clear three hours ahead of me. And there was an attractive riverside walk just behind the house for breaks. I had lived in the area until the age of three and a half, and was sure I had memories of the Atlantic Pond, as seen from a pushchair. As Aidan got used to Suzy, and I knew the sessions would run their full course, sometimes I would just drop him at the house and go on into Cork, to do things, picking him up later.

Suzy remembers Aidan as 'Hawk-eyed, head lowered, but eyes fixed on his subject, ready to pounce, confrontational, interested, very much how I portrayed him in the portrait.'

It was not easy to feel comfortable around Aidan – I think he saw to that – but I did find him amusing, witty, insightful, challenging. I had to take charge during the session, which I think was hard for Aidan, who was a free spirit.

I wanted a mainly red portrait, something dramatic to match Aidan's character. He didn't have red trousers, so he borrowed Joachim Beug's, and we put a red cloth over the chair. He was wary, uncomfortable. He wanted to be back in Kinsale with his work, with 'Zin' as he called Alannah. He told me how he and Alannah got together. He seems to be going through a phase of great anxiety where he frets if she leaves him for any length of time, and has terrible nightmares.

The first half of the session always went like this: Aidan sat dourly, almost glaring at me. I worked away in silence, getting in as much as I could. We worked like this for an hour. I had the presence of mind to offer him a glass of *anís* at the break on the first day – normally, I'd offer tea – but it relaxed him hugely and it became part of the ritual. After his *anís*, he'd drop his guard, and start talking. Anecdote after anecdote, really interesting stuff; material for his books, his life, his sons, his ex-wife, and of course, his life with Alannah. A sort of intimacy developed between us during that time. He asked a lot of me also, demanding to know what made me tick. He liked the way I moved whilst working: walking backwards and forwards from the painting, correcting and checking constantly. He said that I looked like a dancer. I was under a time restraint, so I had to work very hard during the sessions. I had suggested six sessions, and he absolutely didn't want to undertake any more than that.[4]

The painting was almost finished after the six sessions, but still lacked something. Suzy realised what it was:

Mossie the cat: the regal and mysterious Mossie made an appearance in the painting – perched on the arm of the armchair, her stern gaze matching Aidan's. During visits to the house, it was evident that the cats were central to Aidan and Alannah's family, and it felt right to include her. She lends a certain mysterious and calm gravitas to the painting, in contrast to Aidan's unsettling presence. I had to meet Mossie at the house, to make sketches and to get the measure of her, as it would have been impossible to ask for a cat to be brought to my house. In fact, Mossie has a few purposes in the painting: as a commentary on Aidan's and Alannah's home life, as an observer, as a guardian, and as a muse. Mossie was the first animal to be introduced into my work, but animals have since been important to me for symbolic and personal reasons.[5]

The painting was unveiled with due ceremony at a lunchtime event in the Crawford Gallery by the then Minister for Arts, John O'Donoghue, in March 2003.

★

One of the many craft shops that ply their trade in Kinsale during the summer had closed, and by the end of the 2002 had reopened as a bookshop. It had a far better than average selection of books, and Aidan got talking to the man running it. Matthew Geden was an English poet in his late thirties, and had lived in Kinsale for the last few years, while studying part-time for an MA at University College Cork. His wife, Caroline Smith, was teaching at the art school in Cork. They said they were here for good, and could never move back to England now. Matthew was a friend of Desmond O'Grady, and soon he and Aidan were good friends too.

Matthew and a younger local man, Barry Moloney, had published a chapbook edition of some of Desmond's Kinsale poems under their imprint, Anam Press. They asked Aidan if he had a short piece that they could publish. He gave them a choice of three, and they opted for *As I was Riding Down Duval Boulevard with Pete La Salle*, a fast-moving account of Aidan's adventures in Austin, Texas while teaching there in 1984. The photographer John Minihan dropped by one evening on his way home to Ballydehob, and showed Aidan some shots taken on a recent trip to New York. One of them was ideal for the cover of *Riding Down Duval Boulevard*, and John immediately gave him permission to use it.

The little book was launched at Crackpots, the bistro and pottery near our house, whose owner, Carol Norman, sometimes let friends hold events there. Barry told me he and his mother had sat up much of the night before, hand-stitching the spine of the finely produced booklets. There was a large turnout at the launch, and the book sold well. It gave Aidan a much-needed boost after his stay in the psychiatric ward.

The year 2003 was a good one for me as far as work was concerned, but rocky with Aidan. The Health Board psychiatrist was sharp, and apparently enjoyed her skirmishes with him. Eventually she agreed to reduce their meetings to once a month, until they tapered off altogether. As far as I know, nobody ever arrived at a diagnosis beyond acknowledging the existence of a form of mania. 'Mildly bipolar' was the nearest they came, but he seemed to lack the depressive phase of manic depression. Some form of dementia was probably also involved, but apart from Dr Mairead's passing mention, that was not discussed with me again at this time.

Perhaps because he wasn't working on anything, Aidan developed a taste for strong drink that he had not had for a long time, and it clashed with the medication he was still taking for his mental state. Result: sulks, tantrums and what Suzy called 'brattish behaviour'. He also discovered a local source of dope, which led to him spending time with people I described as a crowd of wasters. He became increasingly difficult as the months went by. He started demanding that I help him with his work, specifically that I reorganise his filing system – an impossible chore. Faced with a desk three or four levels deep in papers and notebooks, I honestly didn't know where to start. And every few weeks, even though I was busy with my own work, there was a request for me to type something, urgently. I had already introduced him to a friend who willingly did the bulk of his typing at a reasonable rate, but it seemed there was always something 'urgent' that had to be done immediately.

He especially disliked the fact that, in between stints of journalism, I was working on a novel, and that it was going well. 'How do you know, when everything you've written so far is bad?' He apologised the next morning, and I made a forgiving note in my journal, 'He really doesn't mean to be so demoralising, he just doesn't think – an unusual failure of the imagination.' His birthday that year was the sixteenth we had celebrated together, and his seventy-fourth. We had dinner out at a local restaurant, and it went well. We wondered that the only other two birthdays we could remember were the first one, at which he had accidentally cut my hand with the carving knife while fooling about before carving the duck, and his seventieth in 1997, for which we had invited his ex-wife, his son Julien and two other London friends for a weekend.

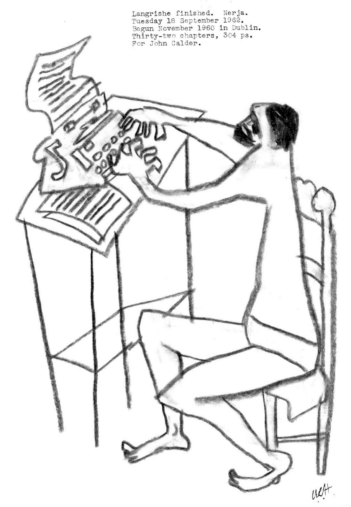

Langrishe finished. Nerja.
Tuesday 18 September 1962.
Begun November 1960 in Dublin.
Thirty-two chapters, 304 ps.
For John Calder.

Self-portrait, on finishing *Langrishe, Go Down* in Nerja, 1962.

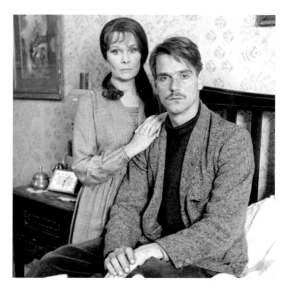

Harold Pinter wrote the script and played a small part, while Judi Dench and Jeremy Irons starred in the BBC's Play of the Week, *Langrishe, Go Down* in 1978. Film still © BBC.

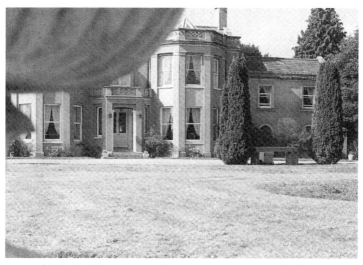

Springfield, the Higgins' family home until 1941, Celbridge, County Kildare. Photograph © John Minihan.

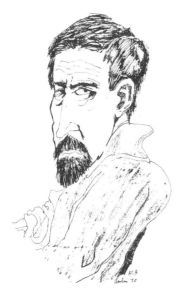

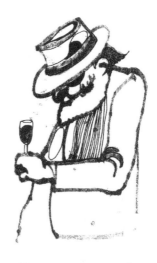

Self-portrait at a Kinsale
drinks party, 1995.

Self-portrait in Berlin, 1971.

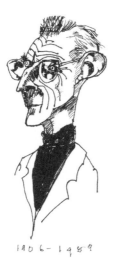

1906 - 1989

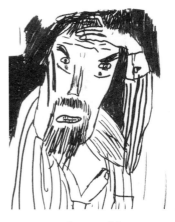

Losing at chess to his son,
London, 1979.

Samuel Beckett, a sketch drawn
by Aidan shortly after Beckett
died, December 1989.

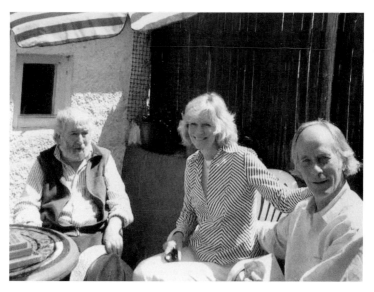

In the sunshine with Kristina Hensley and Richard Ford, 9 June 2007.

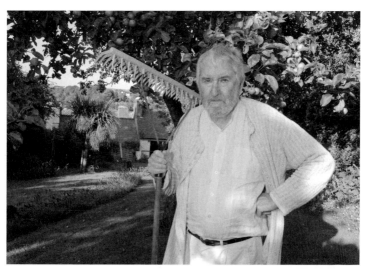

Aidan in his garden, Higher Street, Kinsale, 1997. Photograph
© Billy MacGill/*Irish Times*.

The famously illegible letter written to Aidan by Samuel
Beckett, 6 September 1951. See page 347 for a transcription.
Courtesy of Edward Beckett.

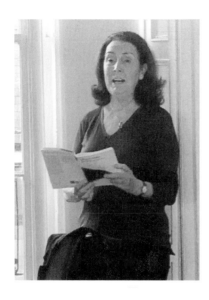

At the launch of my story collection, *The Dogs of Inishere*, at the Origin Gallery, Dublin, 2017.

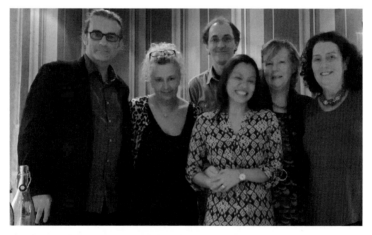

With Keith Hopper, Niamh Moriarty, Neil Murphy and his wife, Su, and Helen Gillard Healy at the Dublin launch of *Writing the Sky: Observations and Essays on Dermot Healy*, edited by Keith and Neil and published posthumously in 2016 by Dalkey Archive Press.

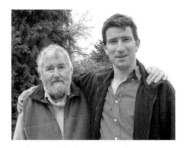

Aidan with his son Elwin,
April 2003.

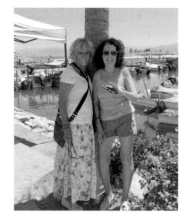

With my sister Pixie in
Mexico, 2016.

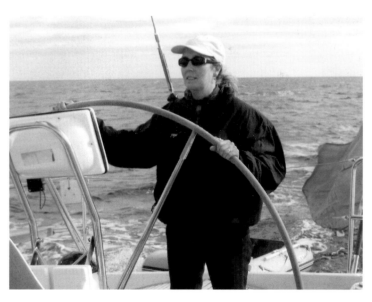

Sailing a friend's ocean-racing yacht back from West Cork.

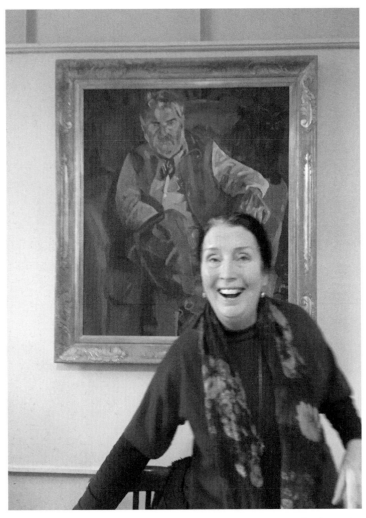

In front of Suzy O'Mullane's portrait of Aidan, Crawford Gallery, Cork, January 2016.

It was a pleasant change to have an ordinary night out. The night before had been typical, me in a bad mood for having written neither a pending travel piece nor worked on the novel, he being argumentative and drinking too much, finishing a half-bottle of Hennessy. I retired to my workroom (the only room in our very small house on which I could close the door, apart from the bedroom), with clinical psychologist Dorothy Rowe's book *Beyond Fear*. I ended up in tears over Rowe's description of borderline personality disorder, which seemed such an accurate description of Aidan. It begins, 'Relationships with others are intense but stormy and unstable ...'

It was seven weeks since I had done any work on the novel. It was not just a question of physical time at the desk, but I also needed space to disentangle my mind from the relentless succession of book reviews, art reviews and guidebook-updating. Long walks and gardening did the trick. By early May a good first draft was nearly finished, bringing an immense relief and an unaccustomed feeling of calm. When it finally went off to Jonathan Williams I didn't mention it again to Aidan.

Work was also going well on the show of outsider art that I was putting together for the Crawford Gallery. I had discovered that several of the more interesting artists in the south-west were self-taught or otherwise originating from outside the usual art school background of most contemporary artists. These included John Kingerlee, an eccentric Englishman living on Beara whose grid paintings and collages were commanding high prices, Tom Walsh, a naïve artist producing highly detailed images of Cork and surrounding areas, and a psychiatric in-patient known as John the Painter. I was given a budget to travel the country looking for work we could borrow for a summer show. My first destination was Tory Island off Donegal, where Derek Hill had encouraged James Dixon and other locals to paint seascapes, St Ives-style. The outsider art project gave me the perfect escape from my increasingly fraught home life.

Talking in Bed

Aidan's voice has started to seep into my consciousness, permeating everything. It begins first thing in the morning, before we even got up. 'Without you, I'm bitched.' 'Do you think I'm selfish?' 'Poor Aidan' – which he knows will bring echoes of 'Poor Cyril', Cyril Connolly's self-pitying moan from a hot bath, reported by his then wife Barbara Skelton. Aidan has many legitimate worries: his fading eyesight, his failing memory, his first two Secker books being remaindered ten years ago (which he still took as a personal insult), and his inability to have full sex any more – a side-effect of his medication. I try to reassure him that it doesn't matter; life has phases, and we should recognise this and learn to welcome changes and adapt to them, not fight against them. Like Cyril Connolly, in a way he too enjoys a good wallow in his misfortunes. There is nothing I can do about any of his problems, except be patient, take him to his various medical appointments and, as Jenny advised when all this began, keep a well-run house with regular mealtimes. I don't cry any more. I have decided that I am beyond crying. Things go in phases. It will eventually get better – or suddenly get worse? No, I have to believe it will get better.

★

I was covering the Venice Biennale for the *Irish Examiner* again, one of the perks of the job. I travelled with a bigger-than-usual group of people because Cork's year as European Capital of Culture was coming up in 2005. I was amazed, while enjoying a canal-side glass of wine on my first evening in Venice, to see an Italian Peter Murray lookalike gliding by, standing in a vaporetto; then I remembered – Peter and his wife Sarah Iremonger were also on the trip: it was the real Peter Murray.

Because Aidan was apparently managing well on his own, I had tacked on a few days to visit Perugia and Assisi. On my way home, I had an hour in Rome's railway station, and spent it choosing a pair of red trousers as a present for Aidan. Unlike Cork city, the boutiques of Rome's railway station had an abundance of red trousers. They were intended as a souvenir of his portrait.

I came back from Italy to a lovely welcome from Aidan and the cats, including an elaborate cartoon of the three of them drawn on a postcard, looking sad and missing Zin. And he was delighted with the red trousers. But within twenty-four hours this had degenerated into the usual harangues: 'don't talk to me about the weather, don't tell me you're going gardening, don't say you'll only be half an hour'. I now have a ring of steel I put up when this happens. I try not to let it get to me, but inevitably something seeps through. He wants me to fight back, and it gets even worse when I don't. His hostility makes me unhappy because I know I cannot put up with this carry-on for much longer, this day-to-day misery, and it's hard to consider the reality of splitting up.

A respite and a truce was declared when I gave him Poem 100 from Augustus Young's *Dánta Grádá*, translations of old Irish poems. It is about lying together quietly on a rug when sex is no longer possible.

Woman who's playful
with me, stay your hand;
wasted is your skill
since I am unmanned.

See my hair is white
and my heart is faint;
what you want to-night
is beyond my strength.

Still don't dismiss me
with an airy shrug
now our bliss can be
only in soul-love.

Though I cannot love
your flesh to fulfil,
on a restful rug
let us play being still.

At least he knows that he is not the only man this has happened to. It is a recurring theme in old Irish love poetry. Can that be what this discord is really all about?

Alannah's Diary, June 2003
Probably I hide too much of my inner life from him, but I've always been secretive. See – there I go, blaming myself. It's what happens after long assaults. But I continue to believe, naïvely maybe, that things will be better. He seems chastened since I went to an afternoon concert at Bantry House with Joachim, and commented on how nice it was to be with someone with such lovely manners for a

change. Joachim drove me there in his Mercedes, we shared a picnic of smoked salmon on brown bread, he looked after me in the interval, and made pleasant conversation with other concert-goers. He even put his arm gently around my shoulder to steer me towards some people he wanted me to meet: it was a long time since I had been treated with such civility. I was well aware that for some people this was the norm; it had once been so with Aidan, and I hoped it would be again.

Aidan is playing with the idea that I really might leave him, at once appalled and rather fascinated, trying it on for size, Aidan alone again. Then he says he likes living with me, and I say, well I like living at home. I cannot in all honesty return the compliment. But neither of us wants to leave our garden, our cats, our workplace or our books. And in spite of all the spats, we still like each other. We are still friends, on a good day, and we will each defend the other unconditionally against any criticism from an outsider. So we must try and find a compromise. The latest one is that he leaves me alone after supper, and goes to bed instead of drinking, so there are no more 'nights of the long harangue'. And also that he does not ask me to type for him, no matter what the emergency. I can be stubborn too.

I had a brief meeting with Jonathan on my way home from Italy. He liked the novel, and thought it was in good enough shape to be sent out in London, after some minor editorial corrections. That gave me a great boost. Apart from a few stories in the *London Magazine* and other small reviews, I hadn't published any fiction since 1985, even though I had been writing steadily. The historical novel had failed to find a publisher, as had a novel about a young Irishwoman in Mexico, based on the piece I had written for Aidan when we first met. 'Beautifully written, but...' was the general verdict. The chief fiction editor of a big London publisher wrote a hilarious letter about the 'beautifully written' Irish-Mexican novel, citing 'ethnic confusion' as her reason for refusing it. So the new novel did not, I hoped, feature any beautiful writing, and neither were there any Mexicans in it. Would that do the trick?

'Irish Outsider Art' opened in early July and occupied the main ground-floor gallery of the Crawford. Aidan was in such a volatile state, and so hostile towards me, that I assumed he would not want to come to the opening. But he was indignant at the idea of being excluded and insisted on being there. It was a lunchtime opening, and I had a tricky-enough cast of artists to look after, both before and after the event, so I asked him to come with Katherine and Joachim. I was worried that he might be disoriented enough to make a scene. He stood slightly apart from the main crowd during the speeches and stood clapping longer than anyone else when I was thanked, until he was the only one still at it. I have never worked out whether this was because he was genuinely pleased for me, or whether he just failed to notice that everyone else had stopped clapping. The show was very popular, and I was glad to have done it. I had hoped it might lead to a book, but there were too many problems with copyright.

*

The Secker books were starting to go out of print. As each book came up for remaindering, Aidan was offered the residue of stock at a special author's discount. There were not many hardbacks left, less than a dozen each of *Donkeys* and *Dogs*, and Aidan bought them all. We were then offered 120 paperback *Dog Days* and about forty copies of a Vintage editon of *Langrishe*. Aidan bought all those too. I excavated some boxes of miscellaneous bits of paper from under his desk, replacing them with boxes of paperbacks. I knew better than to try and argue with Aidan about buying all these books. But I was glad that there were apparently no remaindered copies of *The Whole Hog*, neither hardback nor paperback.

Jonathan Williams was working on a multi-book deal for Aidan with John O'Brien of the Dalkey Archive Press. John had been an admirer of Aidan's work since 1983, when he published a special edition of the *Review of Contemporary Fiction* on his work.[6] Since then, O'Brien had set up a publishing house for the sort of books that he, John O'Brien, enjoyed reading, but nobody, at least in mainstream America, was publishing. He named it Dalkey Archive Press in honour of another much-admired Irish writer, Flann O'Brien, who had published a novel of that name. Aidan was also a great admirer of Flann O'Brien in his many incarnations, and had done extensive research on him while few were interested in his work, making a ground-breaking radio documentary about him.[7]

For twenty years, John had been insisting that Aidan should be considered among the successors of James Joyce, whom he names as, 'Samuel Beckett, Flann O'Brien and – a writer yet to get his fair due – Aidan Higgins, who has some passages of prose that are among the finest ever to have been written in English.'[8]

John came to Kinsale to see Aidan. He had already published the collected stories, *Flotsam and Jetsam*, in a handsome paperback. Now he was proposing to publish Aidan's three volumes of memoirs in one hefty book under the title *A Bestiary*, and to reissue all the fiction that is out of print, starting with *Scenes from a Receding Past*, his personal favourite. We had drinks in the garden, and as John wanted to eat lobster, we went out to a seafood restaurant. Over coffee and cognac, Aidan suddenly dropped a bombshell, and asked John aggressively, 'Why should I allow you to publish my books?' According to John O'Brien, I answered the question, and saved the deal: 'Because he's the only publisher who wants to.'

★

With the coffers nicely topped up by Aidan's first Dalkey Archive Press payment, it seemed a good idea to accept James Hogan's invitation to visit him and his wife, Margaret, still referred to by James as M, in Port-Vendres. He recommended flying to Barcelona, and then taking a high-speed train across the Spanish border to Portbou, where he would meet us. We would be travelling parallel to the smuggling route through the mountains used by so many people over the years, refugees from the Spanish Civil War heading to France, and Jewish refugees fleeing France after it fell to the Nazis, heading for Spain. Portbou, Aidan reminded me, was where Walter Benjamin had killed himself with a morphine overdose, while fleeing the *Wehrmacht*.

We wanted a change from the familiar territory of Nerja and the blandness of the Canary Islands. I was also interested in Port-Vendres' proximity to Collioure on the Côte Vermeille, where the Fauves had painted, and Patrick O'Brian had written his Aubrey-Maturin novels. James assured us that P-V, as its familiars called it, was a low-key, *non-touristique* town, with many good swimming places within walking distance. We chose not to hire a car because I did so much driving at home.

It was an easy journey, arriving in the late afternoon. James drove us to the 'simple hotel' that he and M. had chosen for us. It was very different from what we were expecting: a windowless room in a run-down, dusty place in the town centre, completely deserted, probably used by low-ranking travelling salespeople. James drove off, having told us where to meet for supper.

The dinner went well. M. was a bright-eyed Scotswoman, a biker with a doctorate in Victorian theatre. She was practical and acerbic, the perfect foil to James. She spoke French with a charming Scottish accent, and was starting her retirement by reading every single winner of the Prix Goncourt. She invited me to a *vernissage* the following evening in Perpignan. She thought it would interest me as an art critic to see how they did such things here in France. We would be accompanying her friend the Mayoress, Madame Ginou. Madame Ginou had arranged a *verre d'amitié* in the Centre Culturel to welcome the distinguished Irish writer later in the week, advertised on posters around town. Neither Aidan nor I managed to find a way of mentioning our dislike of the hotel.

Next morning, after a neatly wrapped breakfast – even the croissant came in a cellophane bag – I went to the *immobilier*, and found a suitable apartment. It was owned by Madame Ginou. Port-Vendres, like Kinsale, is a very small town.

That evening Margaret and I left Aidan and James in a bar, with a friend of his, Ian Scott, who had read *Langrishe, Go Down*, and was keen to meet its author. We came back from the *vernissage* about three hours later. Aidan and James had had a monumental falling-out. Aidan had called James a bad poet. James was outside, consoling himself with his pipe, and Aidan was in a corner, sipping brandy and looking shifty. Ian gave us a blow-by-blow account of the evening, which included radical disagreements about Walter Benjamin, Flann O'Brien and Samuel Beckett.

Aidan liked the new apartment, and we stocked up on local wine, which was bought in five-litre plastic containers called *bidons*, and was light and delicious. I went swimming every morning with James, in various wild, rocky coves. We didn't socialise in the evenings. Aidan's son Julien was joining us from Valladolid for the last few days.

Aidan was restless and extremely agitated. The only place that calmed him was the small beach at Collioure. In the mornings he sat in the sun on our balcony, or walked around Port-Vendres. In the afternoons we went to Collioure, sunbathed and swam, and in the evenings we had rows. There was never any question of him being jealous of James; James was simply beneath contempt. In the evenings I attempted to read – Robert Byron's *The Road to Oxiana*, which I had been saving for the holiday – and Aidan, who as usual had not brought any books with him, drank white wine and cognac. His bad behaviour had made me start grinding my teeth in the night, much to my dentist's amusement. Now I was waking early with my brain clenched so hard that it was preferable to get up and walk along the quays in the pale early-morning light than to lie there and seethe. The pointless rows left me defeated, flattened. One morning I woke with a strong visual illusion that I was teetering on the edge of a black abyss, afraid to launch myself into it in case I sank without a trace. Then a strange voice said, don't worry, your friends will hold you up.

Was the abyss life without Aidan? Should I finally decide to leave the venomous toad? Or was it life with him? That night there was a spectacular thunderstorm that left the stone steps outside our first-floor front door churning with rust-red rainwater like a stream in flood. We stood in awe at the sudden force of nature, and watched it, at once fascinated and repelled by the strength of the flash flood. Aidan put his arm around me, as if protecting me and said, 'I'm sorry. I've been an arsehole. A total bollocks.' That's all it took. I knew then that I would never leave him. The real Aidan was not the bad Aidan, the real Aidan was still there, deep inside the other one.

Julien was arriving the next day, and suddenly we very much wanted to be alone, just the two of us. We found him a place in a friendly hostel. Aidan and I were the perfect couple, holding hands and putting on a good show. Pretending it was so helped to make it so: Zin and Moulton against the rest of the world.

Julien was puzzled by Port-Vendres. He wanted to know why people didn't speak Catalan in French Catalonia. I said some of them do, and some of them speak Spanish, but this is France first, and Catalonia second. I suggested that he ask M to explain the Napoleonic Code. When we went to the *verre d'amitié*, Madame Ginou politely addressed Julien in Spanish, as did the people around her. He turned to us with a look of delight, and said 'They're speaking Spinach!' It was the first time Aidan and I had laughed together for months.

★

John McGahern died from cancer, and his funeral took place on 1 April 2006. Since publishing *Amongst Women, That*

They May Face the Rising Sun and *Memoir*, he had achieved an extraordinary level of popularity. Aidan did not begrudge him this, and sent him congratulatory postcards with every achievement, but living at opposite ends of the country, and both being mildly reclusive, they never met again after the conference.

Aidan was genuinely puzzled at the success of *Amongst Women*, the last book of McGahern's he was able to read. Its rural Irish setting and its harping back to Civil War politics struck him as impossibly retrograde. He referred to it as 'twice-cooked cabbage'.

He was equally puzzled by the large number of priests who officiated at McGahern's funeral, and the huge public mourning. He could not understand how McGahern could let himself be buried with such ceremony by the church that had banned his first novel, *The Dark*, had him sacked as a schoolteacher, and caused him to leave Ireland for the building sites of London. I had read that John had agreed to the multiple celebrants at his funeral Mass as a gesture of forgiveness, which I thought very noble of him. But nothing anyone could say would convince Aidan otherwise. Another occasion of Aidan coming over the ridge with a fixed bayonet.

By March 2006 Aidan's hearing was deteriorating, and I often had to repeat things. But what puzzled me was that he seemed unable to use common sense to work out what I was saying. I would remark, walking back from the door with letters in my hands, 'Boring post.' And his query would be 'Boring toast?' When I said 'Five-thirty kick-off,' because I'd been looking at rugby times in the newspaper, he would ask 'Five-thirty peacocks?' I was encouraging him to take an interest in rugby and golf, which he could watch on TV in a local pub, and follow the commentary and the excitement, if not the visual action. I believed that spending so many hours alone in the bedroom in silence, staring at the ceiling with only the cat Naseby for company, was not helping to improve his state of mind.

In late March 2006 I had my own wake-up call. After two rounds of tests, I was diagnosed with a benign ovarian cyst, and advised to have both ovaries removed. I would need six to eight weeks to recover. It was not as drastic as a hysterectomy, but it was major abdominal surgery, and a major logistical challenge to a self-employed writer with an increasingly dependent husband. No lifting or heavy work, and no driving for eight weeks. The consultant, seeing the look of horror on my face, advised me that I should be grateful that it wasn't life-threatening: 'It is almost certainly not malignant. As they sang in Monty Python, "Always Look on the Bright Side".'

I left his rooms in a mild state of shock with the banal little tune ringing in my ears. As if mocking me, on a dark rainy afternoon the lights in the city street twinkled more brightly than normal. As I opened the car door, I leant against the door frame before sitting in, suddenly winded, as if I'd had a blow to the solar plexus. I drove carefully out of town to the car park of Dunnes Stores, then walked around the aisles of new clothes for a while to calm down.

When I told Aidan the news, he asked a very good question, one that I had been asking myself and could not answer: how could someone so active and apparently healthy need such a serious operation? I would have to leave him to manage on his own in the house for at least a week: anything could happen, even with friends to keep an eye on him. I overheard him while he was feeding the cats, 'Poor, poor, poor, poor Zin.'

The first public health nurse I spoke to about getting help for Aidan while I was out of commission was warm and reassuring, but then I was passed on to another, less sympathetic one. She asked numerous questions about Aidan's medical card, which I couldn't find, trying to gauge his entitlement to State care, which is means-tested. 'What exactly would you be expecting the home help to do?' I reminded her that I would be away for at least a week, unable to do housework for another seven, and he was registered blind, and had recently been in the psychiatric ward. He would need help with the cleaning, and also the shopping. She informed me that home helps do not do shopping, the supermarket would deliver. I replied that as she was making it all sound so difficult, perhaps it would be better if we made our own arrangements, and paid for them ourselves. She said again that she would check our entitlements on the medical card and be in touch. Meanwhile, she gave me a forty-page form to apply for carer's allowance.

I told Aidan that I would organise friends to call by while I was away in hospital, and make sure all was running smoothly. His reply was that I must not worry about him, I must worry about myself: he would be fine. It seemed he really cared about me, even though he still seemed bemused about what was happening. But then he had never been very clear about physiology. I was relieved that the self-obsessed gloom merchant I had been living with had disappeared, and been replaced by a much nicer man, warm and concerned. He even suggested that we should go ahead and do some fancy tiling in the hall and bathroom, which we had been discussing for a long time. He thought it would cheer me up.

*

The operation went well, but it had given me a much-needed mid-life shake up. I was now fifty-six years old, and while I had written another two short novels and one long one, none of them had been published. I hadn't published a book since *Inside Cork* with the fledgling Collins Press in 1992. That had been well-received, a true labour of love, but at the end of the day, it was only a guidebook.

I was planning a more interesting book about west Cork, and having been sharply reminded of my mortality, I decided to give it priority, instead of writing fiction that didn't sell. Although Kinsale was home, I am fascinated by that part of County Cork that lies to the west. Ever since visiting it by sea in 1978, I had been drawn to this relatively undiscovered territory with its picture-book farms and cottages, ruined castles, wild headlands and friendly if somewhat eccentric residents.

To hell with the unpublished fiction. The west Cork book was the ideal next project.

Talking in Bed
She: It's no fun being nearly eighty.
He: What's that about atheism?
She: Eighty! No fun being nearly eighty.
He: You don't have to repeat it. I'm not deaf.
She: Oh yes you are. A little bit.
He: Yes, a little bit deaf.

*

An admirer of Higgins called by that August, Neil Donnelly. He didn't let us know in advance, he simply knocked on the door one afternoon and asked if he could borrow a copy of *Bornholm Night-Ferry*. He was a tall man with dark hair, wearing sneakers and a woollen hat, student-like, but too old to be a student. I went and told Aidan, who was as usual lying on the bed, that there was a man at the door looking for a copy of *Bornholm*. It interested him enough to get up and take a look. We went upstairs and had a cup of tea. Neil introduced himself as a playwright and director, and said he had long been interested in adapting *Bornholm Night-Ferry* for the stage or radio. Aidan asked where he lived and he said he was originally from Offaly, but now lived in Donadee, near Naas in County Kildare. I could see Aidan lighting up at the familiar names from his childhood, and soon they were talking of Celbridge, which Neil knew well, Castletown, Killadoon, Donycomper and other local landmarks. He left after about an hour with a copy of *Bornholm*, and I doubted we would ever see him again.

As he made his way home, Neil realised that Aidan would be eighty the next year. As he told me after the event: 'I felt strongly that his eightieth year should be celebrated in 2007 in his birthplace, Celbridge, County Kildare, among his admirers. And so began six months of planning, fund-raising and coaxing Annie Proulx, John Banville and others to take part. It was the beginning of an adventure I was hoping someone else would take, but I discovered that I had no option but to do it myself, because the man's life and work demanded wider recognition.'

*

Aidan no longer took any part in our formerly lively social life, but friends continued to include me in their plans, knowing the situation. He found it very difficult to handle groups, and usually ended up in one-to-one conversation. Then he gradually started dropping his friends, one by one, as his ability to respond to their conversation lessened. He who had once been the liveliest of companions was fading before our eyes. Derek, Joachim, Katherine, Gerry and

Matthew were the last of the regular visitors, dropping by individually every few weeks. All were, in turn, asked by Aidan to cease visiting, until there was only Joachim's long-established weekly visit left.

Whatever I was doing, I tried to be back by six, when Aidan liked to go upstairs and have his supper and perhaps chat, or hear about my day. If I was going to be later, I always warned him, but he didn't always remember, so I never knew quite what reception I would be coming home to. He was constantly on his nerve ends; he called it the heebie-jeebies or the mulligrubs, a term used by Joyce, and hated the prospect of having to see anyone. We devised a system: I gave a short toot-toot as the car passed the house on the way to my parking place, so that he knew I was nearly home, and he had a few minutes to decide whether to get up or not. Valium helped, and I had the GP's permission to increase his dosage as needed.

One evening I was invited to dinner on Heir Island by the Wrixons with the artist Bill Crozier and his wife, Katherine Crouan, art historian and academic, a special treat involving over an hour's drive west, a short ferry trip, an exquisite dinner cooked in the chefs' island cottage, the long drive home, and above all the company, a group of lively and interesting friends. The day before the dinner, Aidan was in such a rage at the idea of me being out for the whole of the following evening that I said, 'If my trip to Heir Island is causing you this much angst, I'll cancel. It's not worth it.'

He turned on me and roared, 'Don't cancel on account of me!'

Then in the early morning I was woken by a monologue about how I was going to come home from Heir Island and find him hanging from a cross-beam in the hall. I had to keep reminding myself that it wasn't the real Aidan, it was an illness. Over breakfast, as if talking to himself, he began, 'We'll get to the point where you can't stand living with me any more and I'll be put away in a home.' He waited for me to contradict him and I said nothing. I was thinking, 'Very likely if this gets any worse,' wondering if he could see into the future. Then he went on, conversationally, 'I can't see out of my left eye. It's all gone dark,' reminding me of the root cause of all this, his loss of sight. I should be more sympathetic. Demons get into him because he's bored, he has a lack of stimulation, lack of the willpower to take himself out for a daily walk, talk to his friends: he could make the decline easier for himself, but he will not.

Zin's Diary, 23 October 2006
Hard to see how it can go on like this, but go on it does. Refused to let him have a kitchen knife in the bedroom 'against intruders'; persuaded him that a number seven golf iron would be a more effective deterrent, so it is installed in the corner. Tension headache whenever I'm alone with him. Hard to know if I'm doing the right thing. Should I be firmer, which only makes him more angry? Should I walk out, if only for 24 hours, or would that make him worse? I am the only entertainment he has, and also the only person for him to get at. Long walks alone on the Old Head beaches whatever the weather are a life-saver. Walks with Gemma, a new, younger friend who is always cheerful, are even better.

Then came the bad news, following a consultation with a geriatric psychiatrist: a firm diagnosis of dementia. I was asked to come and see the GP on my own. He looked at me with such compassion when he told me that tears poured from my eyes. 'The only good thing I can tell you is that it is not Alzheimer's disease, the worst dementia. He will not lose his personality. He has vascular dementia, he will decline in clear steps, and we can prescribe drugs that will postpone that decline. He will be his usual self, only more so.'

Himself, only more so. Dr Mairead said the same, when he had the hypomania. But this is worse, it goes deeper. Logic no longer works, because he doesn't think rationally, and I find this difficult, disorienting. Everything must happen right now. There is no such thing as patience. Sometimes it slips out, I can't help it, at an extreme of frustration I burst out: 'You're acting just like a child!' It is the worst thing I can say. Because deep down he knows something is very wrong, and he knows I know but we never discuss it. That would be impossible.

It helps if I remember to show affection, simple things like hugs and kisses. I hug him more than I would usually, and it pleases him. Must remember to show affection. What kind of a cold bitch makes a note like that?

Good days, bad days, up and down, or down and downer? You are never alone, yet there is no company, no companionship, just his self-absorption. Constant monologues, always the voice, talking to himself when I am not in the room, or to the cats, that are better listeners than I am. Tears this morning in bed, just a little sob, all too much for a moment. Bad. Then I take charge of myself again. No more tears. It happened after I was woken by a sharp kick on the shin: he was fighting in his sleep, dreaming, and thinks I shouldn't hold it against him, because he was asleep. He is right.

I must have no chinks in the armour, leave no crack open through which he can get at me. I think of the village post office and petrol station that I drove past last night, dark-blue shutters pulled down on all its windows, blank, invulnerable. I must make parts of me dead, the parts that he can hurt.

Talking in Bed

Early one morning he tells me his dream of painting a room white. I tell him about the Easter I spent as a student, painting my flat white, bedroom, kitchen, bathroom, hall, white, white, white, and when I wasn't painting white, I was reading Spenser's *Faerie Queene* for an essay. Stately stanzas recounting the adventures of knights, wizards, giants and dragons, and the white-painting created unusually vivid dreams, the best dreams I've ever had. And he remembers a time long before we met, when he too was painting a flat white, several coats of white, and while doing it accidentally hearing Messiaen on the radio, and nothing had ever seemed so beautiful as white paint and the ethereal notes inspired by birdsong. Beautiful white! We cling to each other tightly, in silence, clinging to the rare moment of contact. As in the bad times to come, I will hold on to this memory, the calm and the solace of it, white, white, white.

*

Peter Murray invited me to lunch at the Crawford with John Calder. John was in Cork with his production of *Waiting for Godot*. Before lunch he gave a talk in the lecture theatre to an audience of eleven he described as being of 'Beckettian sparseness', the purpose being to encourage attendance at the play, which was at the Everyman Theatre next week.

Theatre is a new venture he said, because, 'At my age taking on a new author would be like buying a puppy – it's going to outlive you.' John was seventy-eight, a year younger than Aidan. We were at table for over an hour and a half, talk ranging pleasantly over Francis Stuart, Hugh MacDiarmid, the cross-dressing army surgeon James Miranda Barry, when John said suddenly, abruptly indeed, as he tended to, 'If Dalkey Archive want to reprint *Balcony* and *Scenes*, I won't stand in their way. But personally I think *Balcony* and *Scenes* should be re-edited as one book, with the chronology put straight.'

I realised that what I had thought of as a pleasant social lunch had an important subtext. Legally, as long as *Balcony* was technically still in print with John Calder Books, no one else could publish it. Now Aidan could go ahead and sign a contract with Dalkey Archive Press, for a new, re-edited edition of *Balcony*. Outside the Crawford, I escorted John, ever the bibliophile, as far as Connolly's Bookshop, an eccentric emporium selling new and second-hand books, where we parted with a warm embrace.

The news helped to cheer Aidan up, and he agreed to a visit from John and his long-term companion Sheila Colvin. I served a very good white Bordeaux that I had been saving for a special occasion, and John politely commented on its quality. John and Aidan talked of Beckett and his work, inevitably disagreeing: John's favourite Winnie was Marie Keane, whom Aidan thought dreadful. John gave us a programme of his current production of *Waiting for Godot*, and told us that two actors in his company have died so far, one, Anthony Jackson, on stage while playing Estragon. John was backstage calling the ambulance, being asked all sorts of questions. 'Is he breathing?' 'I can't tell you, he's still on stage. Just send the ambulance.'

They parted amicably, with a warm *abrazo*, as Aidan liked to call it, on the doorstep.

*

Neil Donnelly's eightieth birthday celebration for Aidan in Celbridge on 5–6 May 2007 was a triumph of imagination and organisation. The main venue was Celbridge Abbey, where Jonathan Swift had visited Vanessa. We were greeted by a large banner across the entrance, welcoming us to 'Aidan Higgins at 80'. Neil had secured backing from Kildare County Council, the Arts Council and others, and put together a full two-day programme of events. He also produced a sixty-page memorial publication under the title 'A Trade Recondite as Falconry' – Aidan's definition of creative writing. Moreover, Neil had persuaded Annie Proulx, who was giving a reading in the Abbey Theatre the following week, to come over a few days earlier and launch New Island Books' new edition of *Langrishe, Go Down*. Dermot Healy was giving a fiction masterclass, and speaking about the story 'Asylum'. Fintan O'Toole and John Banville discussed Aidan's two Celbridge works, *Langrishe* and *Donkey's Years*, and a symposium chaired by Gerry Dukes with Annie Proulx and Derek Mahon discussed 'Aidan Higgins' Achievement'. Neil wrote and directed two short theatre pieces, 'Jester Higgins', readings of comic Higgins scenes performed by Shane Connaughton and Ingrid Craigie. An excerpt from *Bornholm Night-Ferry*, with the two lovers played by Bibbi Larsson and Denis Conway, was the highlight of the event for Aidan. He spoke ad hoc about his return to Celbridge, commenting that it was almost worth twenty years of neglect for this weekend, and was warmly received. Annie launched the new edition of *Langrishe* with a short but pithy speech, comparing the experience of reading Aidan's work to a quote from Antonio Machado: 'Walker, don't ask where the paths are; you make the paths as you walk'.

On the Saturday we were surprised by an invitation from Libby Sheehy, the current owner of Springfield, to lunch in her dining room. An energetic American, the mother of six children, Libby and her husband Morgan had bought the house in 1989, and converted it into a much-loved family home with large dogs roaming free, and horses grazing in the paddocks once again. Sadly, Morgan died suddenly in 1992, but Libby managed to keep the house on by opening it for bed and breakfast.

It was like a strange dream, to see Aidan and his friends – Gerry Dukes, Neil Murphy, John O'Brien, Jonathan Williams and his partner, my brother Denis and Jenny, among others – seated around the same dining table where he had once hidden under the tablecloth and bitten his brother Desmond's shin, drawing blood. It was very eerie. I had to keep reminding myself this was the real thing, not a film set. I made myself useful helping Libby, who had laid out cold cuts, smoked salmon, cheeses and salads, and even put out the Waterford crystal for us. Annie Proulx congratulated me on being so useful. I don't think she was being sarcastic. I was doing a good job: I genuinely like being helpful when I can.

I was also keeping a close eye on Aidan, without, I hope, intruding on his independence. He had become near enough a recluse, and had trouble both hearing and speaking, and also concentrating for any length of time. A weekend with so many people and events would have been a strain even for someone in the full of his health. But he still had great reserves of energy. In the breaks between events I made sure he had some time on his own, away from his many admirers, to revive, and recover his energy.

He and Dermot had not met face to face since they had fallen out in 1999. Now all was forgiven and forgotten, and it was good to see them having a normal conversation, and parting with the usual bear hugs. On the Sunday evening, a crowd of us had dinner in Barberstown Castle, where some of us were staying with John O'Brien, the publisher of Dalkey Archive, whom we seldom saw. The only one absent was Neil Donnelly, worn out, presumably, by organising such an extraordinary weekend. Aidan was presented with a framed collage of the covers of his published works, which he hung over his desk when he got home.

I spent the rest of that year researching and writing *Eating Scenery: West Cork, the People and the Place*. Most of the work could be done on day trips; I tried not to leave Aidan alone too often, or for too long. He was now on a new anti-psychotic medication, and was much more stable. I no longer had to live with unpredictable mood swings, not knowing if I would come home to a full-blown tantrum, or sweetness. He complained when I had to go out, but also understood that I had to work, and to socialise. For some time now, he had been eating what I called 'a mono-diet' – the same main meal every day. It had been shop-bought quiche for months; now it was shop-bought ready-made pancakes. Both of these I had discovered during my 'decontamination' breaks at Dunnes Stores. It was a boon not having to cook for him.

He enjoyed looking after the cats, which were an endless source of amusement to him. I encouraged him to get out for a walk when the weather was good enough, and he usually went around his beloved Compass Hill – a thirty-minute walk that he would often take an hour or two to complete, as he enjoyed talking to people along his way – neighbours, and strangers, it didn't matter which. In summer he usually wore a Stetson-like riding hat that we had bought in Mexico, which he said turned him into 'Uncle Corn Cob'. Sometimes, if he was getting on really well with people, he would bring them back to the house for a coffee or a gin and tonic – a habit that rather alarmed me. I didn't like coming home to find strangers in the sitting room or out in the garden with him. But somehow, his judgement was sound, and nothing untoward ever happened.

★

In the summer of 2007 Richard Ford was thinking about spending time at University College Cork as a visiting professor. He and his wife Kristina came to stay with our friends Gerry and Marcia Wrixon while they had a look around the area. One morning Richard and Kristina came over for coffee with Aidan. It was a sunny day, so we sat outside on the deck, a small sheltered area behind the house at garden level. They brought greetings from our Mississippi U-based friends, Greg Schirmer and his wife Jane Mullen.

Richard told Aidan that Eudora Welty just stopped writing in her sixties, all of a sudden, because she'd said what she wanted to say. He praised her for being such good company, so interested in all around her, so curious about people. He remembered someone telling her a dream, in which he fell through the sky and landed in a famous New Orleans restaurant, seated at a table, and quick as a flash, she wanted to know 'What did you order?' Then she put it in one of her stories. Aidan enjoyed the talk of Eudora Welty, but was unable to say much because of his aphasia. Nevertheless, he had put together a stack of four Ford books to be signed, two of them hardbacks, and a gift of the new edition of *Langrishe*.

Richard told us how disappointed he was to hear Frank O'Connor's speaking voice in a recording, self-satisfied, talking down to people, 'I thought no, you can't talk like that...' He is a great admirer of 'Guests of the Nation', a fact that Aidan found hard to understand. Aidan agreed with John O'Brien, who sees two strains of writing in twentieth-centry Ireland, the boring and conventional Frank O'Connor followers, and Flann O'Brien's more anarchic crowd.

About a month later (Friday 12 July) we entertained Edna O'Brien on the same deck, rather less successfully. I was looking after her prior to hosting her event at the Kinsale Arts Week. It was the first time I had met her and, like many people, I had been surprised at her old-fashioned County Clare brogue. I remembered Dermot Healy saying after an evening in her company, 'It was like having Mother Ireland whispering in my ear,' and I understood why. She is still very attractive – the red hair, the pale skin, the fine bone structure, the tilt of the head – and beautifully turned out, but at the same time she manages to be very motherly; there is no other word for it. Motherly, but also frail and helpless, making you want to mother her in turn: she cannot drive, cannot swim and cannot walk far due to a foot injury and bunions. But she is very astute, and knows exactly what she is doing. She was also charming, but with a core of steel, interested mainly in herself and her work, and very slightly in other writers of high repute – Derek Mahon, for example, and Aidan – but not the other writers also taking part in the festival.

It was a sunny afternoon, and Aidan, who was expecting us, was upstairs, sitting on the deck. As I opened the front door, I shouted up to warn him I was coming up with Edna. I had warned Edna that Aidan was having problems with his speech, and I left them together while I made the tea. The conversation seemed to be faltering. They really had nothing to say to each other, even in the best of circumstances, but both were being polite, mutually respectful. Books were not exchanged. Afterwards she told me that she envied me, the house, the garden and the ability to swim. I said, 'But you have the whole of London, the theatre, for example.' She replied, 'When I go to the theatre, I am working.'

She gave a wonderful reading at the festival, and was very good with people who came up afterwards to get their books signed, showing a warm interest in them. She said she was useless with money, paying a huge rent every year for her little house in Knightsbridge. From Kinsale she was going to Ballymaloe House for three nights to work on her book about Byron, and I offered to drive her over. On the way she suddenly started telling me about Ernest Gébler, how she still carried an enormous resentment of his discouragement, and about her father's madness. Meeting Aidan had reminded her of these difficult men in her life. She asked me what he was like to live with. I said, 'Aidan has one skin less than most people, he's a redhead like you.' 'I know! I know!' she said, gesturing. She also told me that she knew Aidan was sometimes mad, like her father. 'I saw it in his eyes straight away. It must be very difficult for you.'

Aidan's uveitis seemed more prone to flare-ups in the winter than the summer, or so it seemed as we drove the twenty-seven kilometres to the hospital once again through a dark November day to sit and wait in the Emergency Eye Clinic. There was an operation that might help called an iridectomy, but Mr Murray held this as very much a last resort. There was a risk that any surgery to the eye would set off further severe inflammation, and do more harm than good. But it could also cure the problem. Noting the increased frequency of Aidan's visits, Mr Murray decided to take the risk. Aidan checked in the night before, and I went up the next day, hoping to be there when he came round.

Alannah's Diary, 16 November 2007
Worth the trek up to Cork University Hospital today, the day of Aidan's iridectomy, to see the lovely smile when he woke up and realised that I was there. It seemed like love.

Even better, the operation worked, and there were no more visits to the Emergency Eye Clinic.

*

Early in 2008 Aidan had another small stroke, which affected his speech. He found it difficult to see people without being able to talk to them, and in January he was not up to the usual visit from Joachim, ending a series of almost weekly visits that had persisted for many years. The only good thing to come out of this was a referral to a speech and language therapist. She saw me on my own after her first session with Aidan.

Alannah's Diary, 7 March 2008
A good meeting with Aidan's speech and language therapist Kate, who seems to understand what's going on. She reminded me why she is called a speech and language therapist – speech is one thing, but language, that is to say, communication, is not just verbal, it includes gesture, touch and context. Often Aidan cannot say directly what he wants to say because of the aphasia, but he has

other means of staying in touch. Hence the long monologues in the old days. When I said to Kate it didn't matter if I was awake or asleep or even there at all while he talked, she contradicted me very nicely, and said that my presence was very important to him.

So I am making a conscious effort to touch him affectionately more often, a hug, a kiss on the top of the head, or a squeeze of the shoulder as I'm passing, so he knows I am thinking about him. He has declined so much since last November, since the iridectomy. It is difficult to leave him on his own, but I often have to. He does not always answer the phone, unless it's at 6 p.m., my designated time to ring home, nor can I be sure he will listen to the messages I leave. I worry that he might get into a panic, as he has no sense of time passing anymore, and think I've been away far longer than I have. I worry more about that than I do about him falling. Kate suggests leaving cards with reminders in big letters: Zin away until morning, for example.

The main thing is to carry on, keep cheerful, make him feel loved and valued and safe. I'm starting to sound like a goddamn saint, but it is very important to remember this and act on it. As Montaigne wrote, 'the most certain sign of wisdom is cheerfulness'.

The west Cork book, *Eating Scenery*, was finished, and being edited. Research for the book had brought me into contact with Jeremy Irons. Jeremy had recently spent over a year restoring Kilcoe Castle, a large tower house on the edge of Roaring Water Bay, which had made him a local hero in west Cork, and was duly featured in the book. Jeremy had starred with Judi Dench in the 1978 film of *Langrishe, Go Down*. He and his wife Sinéad Cusack are especially fond of that film, since it was his breakthrough role as a young actor. They were only recently married then, and Sinéad was expecting their first child, so she went to Ireland for the shoot that summer and spent a pleasant few weeks hanging out with Harold Pinter, who had written the script, and also taken a role in the film, which was directed by David Jones. It was shown in the 1990s at Cork Film Festival, with Aidan as special guest, and again on the big screen in 2014 at a gala event in Slieverue, County Waterford, where parts of it were filmed. People who had been extras in the film in 1978, some as schoolchildren, turned up for a gala evening in the presence of Sinéad and Jeremy, who shared their memories in a public conversation. I stood in for Aidan.

Eating Scenery was published by The Collins Press, and was a fine-looking book, with a beautiful cover combining scenery and maps. It was launched in the library at Bantry House in May 2008. Aidan was there with me, and the room was packed with people I knew, many of whom had become good friends in the years since we'd first met.

★

In June, Aidan woke up one morning to discover that he could neither stand nor walk due to dizziness. He was admitted to Cork University Hospital as an emergency. There was talk of a pacemaker, but eventually – over a week later – it was discovered that an adjustment to his medication would solve the problem. He was now taking so many pills that I needed to refill a pill-organiser every week. I was spending ever more time looking after Aidan, and our

GP, Micheál, had advised me to apply for carer's allowance. This would give me enough to live on without working, and relieve a lot of stress. But there was a Catch 22: because I was still working, I didn't qualify for the weekly allowance. Nevertheless, I was given an annual grant towards 'respite care'. The theory was that I would persuade Aidan to go into residential care for a week, which would be paid for by the grant, giving me a break from looking after him. I was so certain that this would never work that I never even asked him. It would have upset him terribly, to be 'put away', while I went off gallivanting. Instead, in a series of ad hoc arrangements, his youngest son, Elwin, and one or more of his four children, kindly came to stay in Kinsale every now and then, while I had some time away.

In September 2008 Aidan suggested that we go to Lanzarote for two weeks in a hotel. With the help of the respite grant, we could travel in style, and so we booked full board in a five-star hotel right on the beach. I was very touched that he would submit to a two-and-a-half-hour flight, and the inconvenience of being away from home, on a holiday that was mainly for my benefit, but he insisted, and we went in late September. Aidan never left the hotel complex, and sadly never found anyone to talk to either, though he tried. He swam in the heated pool, but I couldn't persuade him go out to the sea. He felt safe in the hotel compound and had everything he needed there. I went out every morning for an hour's walk, while Aidan sat by the pool – 'poolside', he called it, as if it were madly glamorous, waiting until I came back to have his dip. One day I forgot to take the hotel key with me. When Aidan noticed this, he decided to go to the back gate and wait there, ready to let me in. On his way, he tripped over a volcanic rock that was part of the poolside décor. By chance, someone was going out as I came in, and I saw Aidan in the distance, stretched out on the ground, his Uncle Corn Cob hat beside him. For a flash second I feared the worst, but once I was beside him I was reassured it was just a minor bump on his forehead, he would be fine. The hotel staff patched him up, but there was no wheelchair available, only a luggage carrier. So he was wheeled back to our room sitting cross-legged on this exotic red velvet platform with a metal curlicue on top. He insisted I take a photograph, and then used it as his Christmas card.

As if I needed reminding, the incident was a confirmation of how frail Aidan had become, and how much he needed looking after. I started reading about the role of carer, for that was what I had become. One booklet advised not to let the person you are caring for take over your whole life: keep valuing yourself for yourself, hold on to your own life. I understood then why I was reluctant to stop working, though I had cut right back.

★

Harold Pinter died on Christmas Eve 2008. Aidan sent condolences to Antonia Fraser, and received this reply:

> *Certainly the last film Harold saw was* Langrishe, Go Down *because it was shown as a memorial for David Jones [the director] at the end of November. Harold was very weak by that time but he was absolutely determined to attend, not so much in honour of David, although he was very fond of him, but because as he put it: 'I've always wanted to see that wonderful film on the big screen.' At the end he felt very satisfied with what, after all, was a cooperative – you, David and Harold.*[9]

I asked Aidan, what is it like to be a survivor? Don't you find it strange that you are still alive and your three brothers are dead, Calnek is dead, and Donal? He said, 'It's not strange that I'm still alive; it's strange that they are dead.'

Colman didn't last long after Sylvia's sudden death. He was diagnosed with cancer, a brain tumour, and was an in-patient for a while, then sent home. He and Aidan were back on lukewarm terms; we didn't visit him. From the occasional letters he sent us – three or four lines – it sounded as if he was struggling. Ye Olde Moncken Holte (as Aidan had nicknamed his house), three miles from the nearest shop, with an open fire for heating and no washing machine, was not an easy house to run if you were physically run down. I had a friend, Sue Leonard, in Ashford, a village near to Colman in Wicklow, and I decided I would leave Aidan for a night or two, and go up and try, with Sue's local knowledge, to find a daily help for him. But before I could get organised, we had a phone call to tell us Colman was in Loughlinstown Hospital, suffering from pneumonia. We should come immediately.

We got there while he was still conscious. He recognised Aidan, and thanked him for being there. He was in a public ward, but was about to be moved to a private room for the night. The young man looking after him was just coming on duty and was very pleased to see us. He didn't think Colman would last the night. He was very upset, and the way he talked about Colman made it apparent that he appreciated his unusual qualities, and the pair of them had become good friends.

We said goodbye to Colman, as it was getting late, and we had to find somewhere to stay. We went into Bray, the nearest town, and all we could find was a grubby room above a back-street pub. We went out for fish and chips, and ate them on the seafront, feeling very sad. The next day my phone rang as we were at a traffic light in New Ross, halfway home. Colman had died.

A letter from the hospital informed Aidan, as next of kin, that there was no need for him to make arrangements: Colman had left his remains to the Royal College of Surgeons. Aidan put a notice in the *Irish Times* to let Colman's friends know that he had gone.

*

Matthew Geden had resumed his visits and was reading to Aidan from 'the Higgins oeuvre' (as Aidan liked to call it) whenever he had an hour or so to spare. He reads very well in a calm tone of voice, with just a hint of his origins in the English midlands. This is Matthew's description of one of those sessions:

> The writer is registered blind. He peers at the reader through thick glasses, blurred vision. He can no longer read his own manuscripts, even when printed large. He rarely goes out now, his world shrunk to a small house in the centre of Kinsale.
>
> 'The dialects of the fishermen here are distinctive, as if they spoke different languages in Scilly, World's End and the Flat of Town. The one-way systems and short interleading streets make the place confusing; you could walk out and come back to what seems a different town....'[10]
>
> And of course it all changes. Houses, roadworks, people on the street. Never the same day twice. The reader pauses, picks up his empty gin glass and walks across to the fridge to pour a refill. The

story told resounds around them, a shared thrill of wandering out of the black Irish night and briefly into the arms of a lost love.[11]

For some time I had been corresponding by email with Neil Murphy, a graduate of NUI Galway, currently associate professor of contemporary literature at the National Technical University of Singapore, who had been commissioned by Dalkey Archive Press to re-edit *Balcony of Europe* with Aidan. He was also editing a collection of academic papers on Aidan, to be published as *The Fragility of Form*, while his colleague Daniel Jernigan was editing Aidan's radio plays. All three books were published in 2010.

Meanwhile, Neil had managed to persuade Cúirt, Galway City's Literature Festival, to give him a slot for an Aidan Higgins event in April 2009. By this point Aidan could hardly see to read, and his memory was totally shot. But he was thrilled at the invitation, and had been writing a paper for the event for four months. Prompts had been typed in 16-point print, which he could read in a strong light. The event was scheduled for the Town Hall Theatre at 3 p.m. On arriving we met Keith Hopper, a friend and college contemporary of Neil's, who was going to conduct the interview. He had reviewed Aidan enthusiastically in the *TLS* several times. We were among friends.

Out on stage, Aidan was quite simply his usual self, but in front of a packed auditorium. Initially, when there was laughter, I was angry, defensive of Aidan, then I realised that they were laughing with him, not at him. The event went very well, in an odd way. Some would call it a disaster, but I liked it because it was just Aidan being himself. When he was stuck for a word, he would look around, blindly, and ask 'Is my wife here? What's that word that I always forget that means "in the time of King James?"'. From the wings I say 'Jacobean'. He can't hear me, but Keith and the audience can, and everyone shouts 'Jacobean!' Then he is answering a question about how he writes, and he can't remember the way Saul Bellow puts it. Again, 'Is my wife here?' and from the wings, invisibly, I say, 'The Hidden Prompter', which brings the house down.

The writer Fred Johnston said afterwards, 'Was the script by Beckett?' which I thought very witty. Aidan's lacunae, and his honest admission of memory blanks, greatly endeared him to the audience. There was a long queue around the bookshop in the foyer afterwards of people with books to be signed. Neil thinks we should do it again in the near future, and have it filmed.

Since I was once again in print, with *Eating Scenery*, I had my own circle of friends whom I ran into on the annual round of festivals. People like Fred, Keith and Neil, as well as Carlo Gébler, who has been a solid friend and supporter since our meeting in 2008 at the Kinsale Arts Festival, Denyse Woods, novelist and director of the West Cork Literary Festival, and Matthew Sweeney, then living in Cork, who had never forgotten Aidan's whispered encouragement before the reading in Belfast. Then there were people I've introduced or interviewed at the Cork International Short Story Festival, or Cork's World Book Fest, or whose books I have reviewed. I have two identities: Aidan's wife, and myself – the Hidden Prompter and Alannah.

*

It was an extraordinary project by any standards, to launch three books at once, so John O'Brien decided to do it in style. Of course, it was not all about Aidan. In the autumn of 2010, Dalkey Archive Press had set up an office in Dublin, and John was discussing various projects with Trinity in both publishing and translation, with complicated issues of co-funding and so on. As far as Aidan was concerned, three of his books were being launched at Trinity, that was the main thing. Ever since he came home from hospital after the stroke, he had been sitting at his desk, making notes for the 'paper' that he would be giving at Trinity.

By October 2010, Aidan was so frail that I thought he shouldn't travel by train, which could involve long walks at either end. In fact, I didn't think he should be in Dublin at all, given his poor state of health, but I couldn't deny him the outing. He had recovered much of his speech, but his worsening memory meant that he often jumped from one topic to another without warning. His wits were scattered. It would be easier to drive up to Dublin the day before the event. Derek, who was to read a poem, came with us. To make it easier for Aidan, I decided we should stay at Buswells Hotel, which he knew and liked, and was only a short walk from Trinity.

By chance, the reading was in the Jonathan Swift Theatre, exactly the same steeply raked lecture theatre where Aidan had read with John Banville and Matthew Sweeney in 1988. But tonight there was an unusual sense of occasion. Neil Murphy and Daniel Jernigan had come from Singapore, the Dalkey Archive people from Illinois, and the room was packed with friends, including Gerry Dukes, Neil Donnelly, Peter Murray and Derek Mahon – Aidan's regular team of supporters.

John O'Brien spoke warmly of his admiration for Aidan, and quoted the ending of *Scenes from a Receding Past*. Neil Donnelly introduced Derek, who recalled visiting Aidan in the hills behind Nerja in Franco's time, and returning there recently, to stay at the Hotel Balcón de Europa. He had been told to read a poem, he said, and he apologised that its title was not original: 'Balcony of Europe'. It can be found in his

New Collected Poems. In it he recalls his earlier visit to 'the novelist', and the comparative prosperity of today's Nerja, where he watched a girl playing on the beach, who in the poem is transformed into the mythical Europa, abducted daughter of the Phoenician king, carried out to sea on a white bull, 'her floaty garments fluttering in the breeze', a translation of Ovid's line '*et tremulae sinuantur flamine vestes*'.

Then Neil introduced his new edition of *Balcony of Europe*, *The Fragility of Form*, a collection of essays about Aidan's work, and the radio plays, *Texts for the Air*. He pointed out how neglected Higgins work is by academics, especially Irish academics. Only two of the essays in *The Fragility of Form* were written by Irish academics, himself and Keith Hopper, neither of whom works in Ireland. A short extract from *Balcony* was read, then Aidan and John O'Brien took the floor for a 'conversation'.

This is Peter Murray's record of the event:

A hunched figure, grey-haired, rises slowly from a seat close to the lectern. Supported by Alannah, he slowly makes his way to the podium, reaching out to support himself, placing his hand against the smooth shuttered-concrete wall. He bends his head close to the book on the lectern, and speaks slowly, with great thought, and with long gaps between some of his sentences.

'John O'Brien … the most elusive of publishers … he publishes a great deal … he is hard to make out, if you know what I mean. He's … you spoke of doubles, we are doubles. From the moment we are born we are doubles. We don't know it, but we are.

John is divided himself. Sometimes he is a grouch, sometimes he is sweet-natured.

I had a fair amount of experience with Calder.
John O'Brien is the easiest man to get on with, once
you get on with him…

I want to read a bit, but I want to see if I *can*
read a bit.'[12]

He did manage to read a little from *Blind Man's Bluff*, which
he had in large print, but it was obviously a struggle. I know
I was not the only one in the audience consumed by pity for
his inability to make out the words. He stopped, and there
was a long silence, then he said, 'Those who want to leave
can leave … it's not the end … but it's the end of me. It's
very difficult to do anything when you are blind. The origin
of the book I am writing now, *Blind Man's Bluff*, is what you
see, or what you imagine you see. When sight goes … it is
replaced by other things … very odd.'

He mentioned his younger brother, who died 'not
so long ago', and from here worked his way around to
Robinson Crusoe. John O'Brien then intervened, to start
the promised 'interview', and they talked about John Calder
editing *Balcony of Europe*. Aidan managed to praise John
O'Brien for 'churning out books'. There was a great surge
of applause, prompted partly, I am sure, by pity. Aidan was
eighty-three years old.

★

Blind Man's Bluff, a small book containing sixty pages of text
and drawings, exists mainly because of the persistence of
John O'Brien. John was keen that Aidan's readers should be
able to enjoy the cartoons and collages that enlivened his
letters, and to read Aidan's own meditations on the trials of
growing old and losing his sight.

By the time that book was being put together, Aidan's dementia had worsened. I had constant requests for typing and retyping of incidents from this book, or for pages to be read to him. At the time I had serious doubts about whether the little book should be published at all, as I did not think it was of the same standard as his previous work. To make matters worse, all the original artwork we submitted was lost in transit in the course of John's many travels. We had copies of some of the material, but not all.

Nevertheless, John O'Brien was keen to go ahead, and now I am glad that he did. The book reads as a record of Aidan losing his sight, as was the original intention, but it also revisits the theme which constantly haunted him: memory, and memory's place in our life as we grow older. I think it also shows that he was aware that his memory and his mind were going, and that he was not going to be able to think rationally for much longer. As such, it is a unique document of mental decline.

If I printed a page in 16-point type, Aidan could read it slowly, letter by letter, word by word, with the help of a low-vision aid that made the most of his remaining peripheral vision. If Aidan had his way, I would be doing nothing all day every day but producing new versions of his latest book. At the time, it was very difficult. Now that enough time has passed, and I am no longer under the pressure I was then, I have come to love this little book, and the insight it gives, often indirectly, in his own inimitable way, to what Aidan was going through at that time.

It is written in short sections, starting with his early memories of Springfield and Celbridge.

The book finishes with two pieces about Robinson Crusoe, a recurrent theme in Aidan's writing since the very earliest days. The parallels between Aidan's loss of memory and words and Crusoe's experience during twenty-eight years of isolation are striking. Who is he describing here, Crusoe and his dog, or Higgins and his cat Naseby?

> Little by little he began to forget his language. It slipped out of his mind, with nothing to read, none to talk to but parrot and dog, his memory grew feeble except for practical matters.[13]

Shortly after the Dublin book launch, Aidan was again admitted to Cork University Hospital after a stroke that affected his speech and his swallow. For a while his vocabulary was reduced to 'No' and 'Bloody Hell'. A friend told me her father had gone through something similar, and the only word he was left with was 'Bollocks!', so it could have been worse. I took advantage of his absence from home to spend a couple of nights on Valentia Island, a favourite escape since my late twenties. Once you leave the main road, it has that special quality of peace that you find only on small islands. I did a lot of walking. In the little graveyard just outside Knightstown I found an inscription on a headstone that read 'I hold you close within my heart, and there you shall remain.' It seemed very beautiful and comforting at the time.

*

It was partly due to the arrival of finished copies of *Blind Man's Bluff* in October 2012 that my inability to provide a safe home for Aidan any longer was finally demonstrated. His behaviour had been increasingly erratic since August. He had lost the ability to tell day from night, and would often get up at 4 a.m. As soon as I heard the shower, I would go and help him in case he fell. He then got dressed, went upstairs, squeezed an orange and had a bowl of bran flakes, then came back and lay on top of the bed until my getting-up time. He had frequent minor falls due to his failing eyesight and his impetuous movements. Once, hurrying upstairs to consult a copy of *Ulysses* for a piece that I was writing, he fell upwards and gashed his head open. He had long since lost his ability to find his way around the town, and would be quite lost only a short distance from his own front door. He had a bulky blue-and-white towelling robe that he wore every day, over trousers and shirt. The neighbours were very helpful. I would come home wondering where he was, and find a message on the answering machine saying, 'Aidan is outside the Blue Haven in his dressing gown and slippers, looking a bit lost'. Thank god for small towns. Sometimes someone who knew him by sight would walk him back to the front door. He never forgot his key, and could always let himself in, having acquired a knack of slipping the key into the Yale lock by feel rather than by sight.

By now he needed twenty-four-hour care, but all he had was me, and an ad hoc roster of friends and helpers. The state provided Deborah for an hour and a half a week. When my GP told them that I needed more help, they added Linda for half an hour a week. Half an hour? It would take him that long to work out who she was. I no longer minded what it cost, we had savings, and we needed much more help than this.

Kerrin and Michael, who had run Aidan's favourite restaurant, Casino House, had closed the business and put the house on the market. Kerrin had retrained as a carer of elderly people, a vocation she had long wanted to follow, and the friend who gave me this news told me that Kerrin might be able to help. It was a godsend; she could give us three hours a week, and Aidan would be delighted to spend time with her. Beside her new qualifications, she had a natural talent for the task, and was a great source of information for me. Matthew continued to read to him whenever he could spare the time, always patient. His equable nature seemed to bring the best out in Aidan. Then there was Belinda, whom we had known since she was a schoolgirl, now the mother of five herself, living only a few streets away, and also happy to help when she could. Then I ran into Pat O'Mahony, our former hairdresser, whom I hadn't seen for years. She had also retrained as a carer, and said to call her if I ever needed help.

I had to go to the west of Ireland for three tightly scheduled days and nights on a guidebook recce, and drew up a roster of helpers. I felt bad at having to leave Aidan, but the trip was essential, and would bring in a much-needed big cheque. I felt it should be possible.

I spent the first day in Galway city dealing with a list of hotel and restaurant visits. The next day I headed out to Connemara, and my spirits rose almost to holiday mood as I drove west. As always, the mountain scenery and the big skies were soothing. We had recently watched *The Quiet Man* on my iPad, and as I drove past the sign for the Quiet Man Bridge I remembered Aidan's enjoyment of the familiar scenes and dialogue. I had to visit a new place, a Celtic-themed garden designed to entertain both Irish children on school trips, and grown-up visitors in search of Celtic mythology. When I arrived, I went for a coffee while a shower passed over, and I finally started to relax. Instead of criticising the simple 'Celtic' theme, I decided to go along with the spirit of the place, as if I were a real visitor, not a researcher on a quick recce. One of the unusual features was an indoor tree, whose 'leaves' consisted of hand-written messages to loved ones, alive or dead. I took a piece of paper and wrote, as if by automatic hand, 'For dearest Aidan, may your soul soon find peace', and attached it to the tree. The moment suddenly threatened to overwhelm me, as I realised how frail Aidan had become, how close he perhaps was to the end, to death, and how little he or I were able to change anything. I stood and stared at the tree for a long time, feeling simultaneously a great sadness and an enormous relief, like the lifting of a burden. I knew Aidan and I were coming to the end of a phase, but I had no idea what lay ahead.

★

There was great excitement as always when the first finished copies of *Blind Man's Bluff* arrived. It is an unusual and very attractive little book, and was the first time Aidan's drawings had been included in any of his own books. Matthew had the idea of putting on a display of Higgins' 'oeuvre' in his bookshop window, displaying the Dalkey Archive editions and New Island's edition of *Langrishe*, with *Blind Man's Bluff* as a centrepiece. That Monday, we collected drawings, collages and photographs, and I walked Aidan down to the bookshop, where he spent the morning with Matthew, doing up the window. I brought him home for lunch, and while he was resting afterwards, I went to my desk in the front room to do some work. I was disturbed by a fracas outside my window. A car had stopped in the middle of the road, and its driver was bent down in front of it. When I opened our front door, I saw Aidan stretched out on the road, clutching another batch of material for Matthew, the car only a metre or so below him. He had tripped and fallen, while sneaking past my window to make a solo excursion to the bookshop. He found it funny rather than alarming, to be lying at full length in the middle of the road in front of his house. He had a minor bump on the head, and a sore arm.

The pain from the arm kept him awake all night, so next day we took him for an x-ray, and a cast was put on his broken arm. This proved to be too tight, and after another sleepless night we went back the next day to have it adjusted. While I was asleep that night, Aidan picked the whole cast loose, and removed it. By Friday he was so agitated that we were back to the GP, who recommended increasing his dose of Valium as a temporary measure, and took a urine sample, the result of which we would get on Monday. Two more sleepless nights followed on Friday and Saturday, with Aidan continually up and down the stairs, hallucinating and disoriented. First thing on Sunday morning, I phoned the emergency GP service, and also our friend Pat O'Mahony. Eventually, after Pat had been there long enough to assess the situation, our friend David Nagle, the head of the practice, arrived. Luckily he just happened to be the GP on call. His presence had an instant calming effect on Aidan. All of a sudden they were sitting down, David holding both Aidan's hands in his, having an apparently rational conversation. He persuaded Aidan that it would be a good idea to go into Accident & Emergency and see what they could do to make him more comfortable. While I had been assuming he would be admitted to the psychiatric ward again, David explained that he suspected an underlying cause for the agitation. Most likely the psychosis had been brought on by an undiagnosed infection. If he had an underlying medical condition, he would be admitted not to the psychiatric ward, but to a normal medical ward, while the cause of his condition was investigated. Pat sat with Aidan in the back seat of the car, for safety sake, while I drove him to the hospital and we took our place in the waiting room at A&E.

Late in the afternoon of 28 October 2012 Aidan was admitted to Cork University Hospital. A medical orderly was stationed beside his bed to calm him when he tried to get up. He needed twenty-four-hour supervision. Reluctantly, I left him on the ward and returned to the silent house.

Aidan never came home again.

PART IV
Scenes from a
Receding Life
2012–15

From early October 2012 Aidan was an in-patient in a general medical ward for more than six weeks. His case was typical of many others: the medics and the bureaucrats had agreed that he should not be discharged back into my care, he should go to a residential home where he would have twenty-four-hour supervision. We had done the paperwork: he would qualify for something called the Fair Deal: in return for 5 per cent of our assets, I would be allowed to continue to live in our house, and all Aidan's income would be used to pay for the nursing home. There was only one hitch: we had to find a home that had a vacancy, and was willing to offer him a place. Meanwhile, he stayed on the medical ward in the big hospital.

A place came up at a home not far from Kinsale, and my spirits rose, but they turned him down. They said he was 'too agitated'; they feared he wouldn't fit in. I reckoned what they really meant was that he would be difficult. I was now considering places within an hour's drive of home, including the place in Clonakilty where Kerrin was now working.

Meanwhile, he was hating the six-bed ward where he had already spent a month and a half, and I was devastated to see him in this limbo, angry at being confined, desperate to escape, but unable to understand why he couldn't go home. The cause of his psychosis turned out to be a urinary tract infection, and it was cured by a course of antibiotics. His teeth had also been looked after, and the psychiatrist he had been seeing as an out-patient had a long interview with him. They were still trying to fathom his 2002 suicide attempt, and see if they could find anything to add to the diagnosis of dementia.

Whenever he could, Aidan would make a run for it, and the security guards had to be constantly vigilant. There was usually a radio playing on the ward, which irritated him greatly, and he would regularly ask for it to be switched off. One afternoon it all got too much; he picked it up and threw it out of the third-floor window. I was secretly rather proud of him, and the nurses were smiling too.

Christmas was getting nearer, and it looked as if he would be stuck in the hospital for the holiday. One day a woman called Julie, who looked familiar, came to visit him from Ballintobber Lodge, an old country house in its own grounds, not far from Kinsale, that had been converted into a nursing home. It turned out that Julie was familiar because she had been the ward sister when Aidan was admitted to Cork University Hospital, six long weeks ago. She had been working for an agency then, and had quit to become the nurse manager at Ballintobber Lodge. She was a warm, intelligent woman of retirement age who didn't want to retire yet. Soon after her visit, I had a call from the unfortunately named 'Discharge Co-ordinator': Ballintobber Lodge was offering him a place; would I like to go and see if it would suit him?

I was so overwhelmed by this stroke of good fortune that I had to struggle hard to keep back tears of relief as Julie showed me around. I had been to the house once before to visit a neighbour from Summercove, a bachelor who had become unable to look after himself. It had also been the place where my mother's friend Joanna Good had spent the last six months of her life. Since then a lot of the trees that had overshdowed the place and given it a reputation for being gloomy had been cut down. A sunroom had been built on to the front, and another added in the centre of the ground floor, which led out to an enclosed garden with a large fishpond. I was told that Aidan would have to share a room initially, but when a single room became available, he could move. His room would have been the master bedroom in the nineteenth-century house. It was at the top of a splendid wide staircase, above the front door, and had three French windows facing south-west. It was uncannily like his mother's bedroom in Springfield. There were two other occupants: a relatively young man with an intellectual impairment, and a retired fisherman whom I knew by sight from Kinsale. It was perfect. It was also very sad. But there was no other choice. He simply could not live at home any more. As I thanked Julie, the tears came down. It was 21 December. 'Why don't you go away for Christmas? You need a break. He'll find it easier to settle in if you don't visit for a while.'

So I booked a flight to London, and a room for three nights at the Airport Hotel in Croydon, as my brother's house was already full. To give some idea of the state I was in – I booked a flight to Stansted, not Gatwick. When I got to Cork airport, I thought I'd better tell the people at Ryanair that they had put the wrong destination up: this flight was going to Gatwick, not Stansted. When I realised my mistake, I was so flustered that I couldn't remember how to dial my brother's London number on my mobile; at home I had it keyed into my landline. I had to ring a friend in Kinsale, and ask her to ring Denis and tell him I would be late because I was flying to the wrong airport.

When I got back to Kinsale and started visiting Aidan in Ballintobber Lodge I got into the habit of making notes afterwards, to help me to make sense of this new routine:

13 January 2013

On arriving to see Aidan today he made me write down 'My anguish is not very good,' words of the departing laundry maid, who had in fact said, 'My language is not very good,' meaning her English.

29 January

Good weather on way back from Killarney, so went up to St Gobnait's graveyard in Ballyvourney to walk among the tall trees and visit the three Seáns: Seán Ó Riordáin, Irish language poet, Seán Ó Riada, the musician, and Seán Dunne, a friend and contemporary. I made a note of the inscription: 'Seán Dunne Poet 1956–1995. In the beginning was the word. In the end there is silence.' I thought of Aidan, already well along on his voyage to silence.

Daily visits to Aidan were a strain for both of us. Julie suggested I make it every other day. Then one day as I was leaving he asked will you be back again tomorrow? I said, 'Yes, of course.' Feeble.

He was in low spirits and disoriented. He was in despair of ever getting out, asked if I'd tried John and Nuala Mulcahy again and Fintan O'Toole at the *Irish Times*. He believed he had been kidnapped and detained against his will, and wanted me to let his powerful friends know his situation. When I took him out to the garden he howled, and cried and said, 'My mind is going.'

Back in his room, he couldn't follow the new chapter of *Dog Days* I was reading to him; he wanted yesterday's chapter about Blackie again. Why not?

Later I learnt that his ability to understand what I am reading to him fluctuates from one visit to another because of the physical source of his dementia. With vascular dementia, the flow of blood to different parts of the brain can vary from one day to another, affecting mood and inhibitions, and also, apparently, comprehension.

13 February

A bad farewell, Aidan wanting me to stay on and read to him. He's lying on the bed saying, 'You have no idea what it's like to be old and alone,' and tearing his hair. Then hardly is my back turned, before he's trotting downstairs for a nice cup of tea. I know, because Julie told me when I went back in from the car park, unable to leave him in that state.

I discover that my friend Gemma spent a lot of time looking after her grandmother, and worked in an old folks' home one summer as a student. She says it's a well-known phenomenon, the residents put on a big show of hating it there when they have visitors, and as soon as the visitor has gone, they are right as rain again. I can believe it. The past week has been much better, I go down earlier, about 11.30, and stay an hour. Then when I am leaving, he has the distraction of lunch. His lunch is served in his bedroom because he doesn't like eating in the communal dining room. 'Who are all these old people? I have nothing in common with any of them.' I like the management's kindness and flexibility.

I'm still having trouble with the junior doctor who seems to think Aidan is perfectly well and fit to be discharged home. The only reason he isn't is that I will not agree to look after him. This is a distortion of the facts: he needs 24-hour supervision for his own safety and that of other people, including me. I will fight tooth and claw for him to stay where he is, and I know the senior docs will support me. Even so, I am very anxious.

Then I was encouraged by Matthew saying unprompted, 'But he's doing so well at Ballintobber Lodge. If he comes home, he'll regress.'

I called into Ballintobber Lodge for an hour most days, as early as possible after 11 a.m. I never visited after 4 p.m., because I thought it good that Aidan knew not to expect evening visits. I imagined it would help him to settle down, and agree to go to bed.

There were good patches and bad. He enjoyed his interaction with the people looking after him, the Polish woman who brought his clean clothes, the lovely blonde Eimear who brought his lunch, his face lighting up when she said, 'Turkey!' (his favourite) and 'Ice cream!' Whoever dressed him in the morning, usually Rollo, took great care to add a silk scarf, loosely tied at his neck, and to shoot his cuffs out from under his sweater.

But there were still days when he was obsessing about getting out again, and I was greeted with, 'What do I have to do to get out of here?' 'Let me get in the car now, and go.' I recognised the feeling from boarding school, and it upset me too, that he had to be confined. If his pleas went on, and often they did, on and on, I stopped visiting for a few days. Gemma gave me that tip. When I reappeared, he was like another person, all sweetness – forgetful, a little confused, but happy with the people around him, and grateful for whatever I had brought – flowers from the garden, or a Kit Kat. Some days after lunch, the young ones played his music – the Gypsy Kings or Bob Marley – and danced with him.

Carmel, who was in charge of the social calendar and entertainment at Ballintober Lodge, tried to interest Aidan in audio books, as he can no longer read. He explained that for him reading is a silent activity, and he does not like the idea of *listening* to a book, especially not if there are actors involved. He spent a lot of time when working on radio plays sourcing actors who did not sound like actors. (Norman Rodway was his preferred choice as narrator, and he did sound uncannily like Aidan.) But he agreed to have a go, to please Carmel. It turned out that the only name on Carmel's list of writers available in audio books that he knew (apart from Maeve Binchy) was Ernest Hemingway. 'We'll give it a lash,' she said, and he loved that. 'We'll give it a lash,' he repeated, laughing. It was good to see him making another friend in his new world.

*

I took on a Writers in Schools course, two hours once a week for six weeks. Going into schools sharpens you up, and it is always fun to introduce the teenagers to the kind of writing that contradicts their expectations. But I had had to stop taking on these occasional, well-paid jobs, because while Aidan was still at home I couldn't rely on being able to turn up somewhere at a particular time, calm, neatly dressed and well prepared. It was good to be back in the old routine.

7 March 2013

Aidan has been in the home for ten weeks. Today he was not sure who I was until I told him, which was a shock. I read to him more slowly than usual, and I noticed that he is having more trouble than usual talking, finding the words. Kerrin is busy moving house, but she kindly came to see him when I asked, a friendly call; she would not hear of being paid for her time. She says his aphasia is getting worse, but there is probably not much that can be done about it. It is consoling to know that even if I had unlimited funds, there would not be much more that I could do to help him. Age is taking its toll, and the damage cannot be reversed. He was delighted to see Kerrin, and made a big fuss of her.

I brought him a DVD of *Citizen Kane* and we went looking for someone who could work the DVD player on his TV. (After all those years of not having a TV, I am a total dunce with a zapper.) For the first time he was greeting the other oldies that we met in the corridors with real affection, warmly shaking their hands, 'The man with the cap!', another old man with a stick asks, 'Is this your grand-daughter?' That cheered me up. He told the huge fat man in an armchair at the kitchen door that he had Orson Welles in *Citizen Kane*, and showed him the DVD. Then he went back alone to his room to wait for the charge nurse to come and put it on – there was no problem at all with me leaving. I saw him waving from the bedroom window above the front door, always a good sign.

I can love him again now that we are not in daily battle over small things, now that he is not tormenting me with his demands. I admire his warmth and generosity towards other people, his unique and strange way of relating to people. Long may it last.

Two people in the past week have told me I'm looking more like my mother. I take it to mean I'm looking older, my face is sagging, and I've put on weight.

Why do I take it like that? Why not assume they meant I'm looking beautiful and kindly – as people say my mother did?

Rosita, a former girlfriend, came down by bus from Dublin on a sudden impulse, dressed as if for a cocktail party. Suzy O'Mullane, who is a friends of hers, came over and they visited Aidan together. Suzy had very cleverly worn bright-red high-heeled shoes, hoping the red would remind him of the portrait. He referred to her as 'the artist', so presumably it worked. The staff were intrigued by these two exotic visitors.

I had a text from Rosita the next day – she and Suzy had talked and talked about me and Aidan, and the huge amount of sadness I was living with; she called it 'the heavy burden of sadness'. I woke in the night and made this note: 'Don't feel it as sadness, turn it into love.'

That made sense: the sadness comes from compassion for his confusion and his inability to understand his situation, and compassion is the obverse of the coin of love.

6 May 2013

Pat Cotter, the director of the Munster Literature Centre, has suggested that I give a short story course at UCC in September as part of the Cork International Short Story Festival. It will also be an option on UCC's inaugural Creative Writing MA. I met the new head of English, Claire Connolly, today, and she agreed to the idea. Pat tells me I am lucky to get it. He says it is hard for him to give me all the work he would like, because I haven't published a collection of stories yet. So I will have to do something about that.

I went to Debenham's to buy an outfit to wear to a wedding, and found something suitable in the sale. So I blew what was left of the budget – €80 – on a swish new carry-on suitcase, dead smart, acid green with four wheels, a lock and a five-year guarantee. I shall be travelling again, now that Aidan is being properly looked after. As I got out of a traffic jam and accelerated up the airport hill, I heard the chorus of the huntsmen from *Der Freischütz* on the car radio, and had a repeat of the euphoria that I had the first time I heard it from my seat in the stalls at Covent Garden, the jaw dropping, head buzzing with pleasure at the discovery that opera could be this much fun.

Later on I wondered how I could let myself be so happy when Aidan is so miserable. But is he really?

Tomi and Yvonne Ungerer came on a visit. I met them outside Kinsale, and they followed my car to Ballintobber Lodge. They were spending the night in the airport hotel before an early flight to Switzerland, en route to Alsace. Yvonne looked wonderful as always, a tailored tweed jacket, long black hair worn loose. I took them up to Aidan's room. He was delighted to see them, and had a notion to take them out to Jim Edwards' for a meal, and then home to the garden. Aidan and Tomi sat on a wooden bench in the garden, and we were all given a glass of wine by the young manager, who could see this was a special occasion. I took some photos, and Tomi was delighted because he wanted a photo of himself and Aidan for a tin that he takes everywhere with photographs of all his friends in it. I told him how much I liked *Vracs*. He was pleased with it too, and on the strength of that book, he has been given a regular page in a French philosophy review: he, who had never even passed his baccalaureate. He said, apropos of something else, 'If I can be blunt.' I said, 'Although you are very sharp, Tomi', at which he whipped out a little red Silvine notebook and jotted it down, 'I am blunt and I am sharp'. Yvonne said she was tired after nearly three hours' driving. I asked why it took three hours and, quick as a flash, Tomi, who doesn't drive anymore, answered, 'Because *she* was driving.' Yvonne countered by saying Tomi should never have learnt to drive: 'You cannot imagine the horror of Tomi taking the highway from New York to Long Island on a Friday evening...' Tomi was comparing ages with Aidan, 'I am eighty-two, that is not my age, it is the speed at which my life is passing, and Aidan is going even faster at eighty-six.'

*

It took me a long time to get used to having my freedom back: I had such richness of choice – to walk the Old Head beaches, or the waterside footpath from Charles Fort to Lower Cove, or both if I liked. No one was waiting for me at home, fretting that I'm still out, getting angry at perceived neglect. The cats slept peacefully, and woke and stretched silently when I came in. And when I was home, I was free to have the radio on, or play music. I could read the newspapers without being criticised for wasting time, stay out gardening as late as I like. I could even watch the television news, for after some thirty years without one, I had bought myself a TV set. I spent much of the first year that Aidan was in Ballintober Lodge gently thawing out, getting used to normal life again, the simple pleasures, the greatest of which is solitude. It was a long time since I had had that much peace and tranquillity.

I heard from a friend who did art therapy at Ballintobber Lodge that Aidan was really happy there, and everyone loved him. Some weeks were more difficult than others, and I worked hard at cheering Aidan along, reading to him, even though his comprehension was shrinking. Sometimes it seemed he didn't hear the words any more, just the sound of my voice, the way it happens when you are about to fall asleep while someone is talking, like in the back seat of the car as a child.

*

When I met Aidan I was going through a flirtation with Catholicism, the religion I was born into and brought up with. The attraction persisted on and off for a long time, but was finally nailed during what I call 'the bad Aidan years'. There were times when I was in deep despair at having to live with someone so difficult, while also trying to have a life of my own and keep cheerful. It helped that I didn't necessarily assume that everyone is entitled to an easy life. You are not going to be happy all the time. Inevitably there will be rough patches, so you find a way of getting through them. Cultivating a habit of gratitude, which was popular among the self-help crowd at the time, turned out to be a way of avoiding troughs of despair. So was mindfulness, learning to live in the moment. When I was at a particularly low point, a friend who was also looking for ways through a bad time told me that the services at the Baptist church in Kinsale were very good. While I was not up to going to a service, I wandered into the church one Sunday morning and picked up a tiny publication about eight centimetres square called *The Little Book of Help*, free to take away. It consisted of short quotations from the scriptures, grouped under headings – money, ambition, friends, sex, attitudes – nicely laid out on the page like poems, with plenty of white space. Some of them really did help:

> If you are cheerful,
> you feel good;
> if you are sad, you hurt all over.
> – Proverbs 17:22

> Ask, and you will receive.
> Search and you will find.
> Knock, and the door
> Will be opened for you.
> Everyone who asks will receive.
> Everyone who searches will find.
> And the door will be opened
> For everyone who knocks.
> – Matthew 7:7–8

You really do have to learn to ask, and when you ask, it is surprising how much you are given. Not asking ensures that you stay miserable.

Encouraged by this foray, a few weeks later I ventured into the Catholic Parish Church on a similar quest, and picked up a little publication that turned out to be the worst kind of pro-life propaganda. I was looking for spiritual help, and they gave me anti-abortion rants. I have not prayed as a Catholic since. Not for me. In fact, I gave up praying altogether, just when I probably needed it most. But it felt better, and more honest to soldier on, godless.

The last books that Aidan read before his eyesight finally gave up were Antony Beevor's on Berlin and Stalingrad. He had long had an interest in Nazi Germany, since childhood I imagine. He had a well-worn copy of Albert Speer's *Inside the Third Reich*, and Gitta Sereny's lengthy biography of Speer. He was definitely fixated on Speer, though he never wrote anything substantial about him. But he often told the story of Hess's imprisonment, the changing guards, his garden and the visits of his wife.

At Ballintobber Lodge, the book he most treasured was *Tomi: A Childhood under the Nazis*, Tomi's childhood memoir of growing up in Alsace. Neither Tomi nor his mother ever threw anything away, and the book is illustrated with a wonderful array of family photographs, childhood drawings and Nazi memorabilia sent to him by readers of the French and German editions that preceded this English one. With his remaining eyesight, Aidan could pick out many of the illustrations, and enjoy them, as if they were discovered afresh every time. There were certain passages that he loved having read to him again and again, including one in which a German officer talking to his mother admires the row of chestnut trees:

'Are they not beautiful at this time of year? One thing I promise you: the day will come when you will see a Jew hanging from every branch.' Then he pulled out a piece of paper. 'This is a wonderful recipe for carrot cake. My wife gave it to me – it is yours.'[1]

Another favourite was a Taschen edition of the works of Matisse, which he loved for its colours and the bold shapes. He could sit on his own, and gain some pleasure from just flicking through its pages.

He also enjoyed a group biography of Cyril Connolly and *Horizon*, the review he edited – *Friends of Promise* by Michael Shelden. It is hard to believe now, looking at the dense print, but between us, Matthew and I read the whole book aloud to Aidan, and he seemed to revel in the detail: 'In 1940 Cyril Connolly's father, a retired major of the King's Own Yorkshire Light Infantry, sent his son a thank-you note for the latest issue of *Horizon*, the first he had enjoyed reading...'

I went to Mallorca for a week in mid-June, mainly because I could. The Mediterranean sun and sea were wonderful, and friends recommended good places on the Tramuntana coast. I visited the monastery where George Sand stayed with Chopin and sent Aidan a postcard. But I was appalled at how heavy and unfit I had become in the past year, and resolved to do something about it. Back home, I got into the habit of walking for at least an hour a day, and felt much better. As soon as it was warm enough, I started swimming in the sea most days, usually with Katherine or Gemma, and life was good.

5 December 2013

Some times when I arrive I see Aidan has put his books together neatly in a pile, Tomi Ungerer's *A Childhood under the Nazis*, *Dog Days*, the Cyril Connolly biography, and a notebook he sometimes draws in, and I know these books are ready to go home with him, and he is going to mount a 'take me home' plea.

Other times, when we have a good visit, and enjoy each other's company, say he laughs at what I'm reading, then he suddenly bursts out with, 'Why can't you take me home, now?' Because we've been liking each other, he expects me to be complicit with his plans to escape. Another day he was highly excited when I arrived, books under his arm, 'We'll get in the car and go straight to the bank, take out all my money, then we'll go to the airport and take a flight to Lanzarote. You like Lanzarote.'

Today, before we got to the 'take me home' plea, I made a big effort to explain to him why I can not take him home: 'It would be dangerous. You are not getting enough blood to the brain...' which only sends him into a rage: 'You are cruel, cruel...' Any logical argument is anathema to him, presumably because he cannot follow it. The nurse manager heard the roaring, saw my face and suggested I stay away for a few days. 'Don't feel guilty, it's the best thing to do. You are his only reminder of home, it brings it all back. He will have forgotten in ten minutes. I'll go up and see him and talk about something else, and he will be perfectly alright.'

It is almost beyond my comprehension to grasp the fact that Aidan cannot, and never will understand his circumstances. Kerrin has already explained to me that when he asks to be taken home, he is expecting me to rescue him from his prison of incomprehension, his cloud of doubt and uncertainty, take him back to how he was before he fell ill. Because I refuse, and say I can't, they won't let me, he accuses me of being cruel and evil. Of course he does. To him it makes sense.

It never fails to touch me, his simple faith that by doing the right thing (whatever that may be), like a little boy, he will be rewarded by his freedom. 'What do I have to do to get out of here?' But as Kerrin says, what he really means is 'What do I have to do to be well again?' – able to live independently, and make my own decisions.

One day in summer of 2014 I was walking through Waterstone's and a large-format children's book caught my eye: *Moon Man* by Tomi Ungerer. Designed to be read aloud to very small children, its densely colour-saturated illustrations were ideal for someone with very little eyesight. The man in the moon leaves his seat in space, and catches a lift on a passing comet to visit the people on earth and have fun with them. But because he glows and is strange, he is taken for an invader and thrown into gaol .... It was lovely to watch Aidan's total absorption in his friend's fable.

Before Aidan's long stay in Ballintobber Lodge, I would have assumed that everyone in a residential home was beyond finding pleasure in everyday life. It was humbling and very moving to learn otherwise. The simplest things can give great pleasure: there is a different quality of life, but it can still be savoured and celebrated.

There were many visitors during the three years that Aidan spent in Ballintobber Lodge, young and old, and I was very grateful to all of them. People who hardly knew him came and read to him, or took him out for a cappuccino in a nearby pub. But other friends and relations were not up to visiting him in a home, and I completely understood their reluctance. Everyone did what they could, whatever they were comfortable with. Aidan was always delighted to see people, especially younger people, and gave everyone a big welcome.

During the third Christmas that Aidan spent in Ballintobber Lodge, Christmas 2014, I stayed in Kinsale, but I didn't visit on the day itself, when a festive lunch was provided for the residents, and they were given individual presents. I spent the holiday reading Atul Gawande's book *Being Mortal: Illness, Medicine and What Matters in the End*, and never was time better spent. Gawande is a surgeon in Boston and a staff writer for the *New Yorker*, and his book is about growing old, and how we care for the elderly in affluent Western societies. His book is essential reading for anyone trying to help an elderly friend or relative negotiate their final years of life. According to Gawande, nursing homes like Ballintobber Lodge, ones that are friendly, flexible and above all kind, are far preferable to well-regimented, high-tech homes, which are often run as much for the convenience of the staff as for the well-being of its inmates. I was glad that we lived in rural Ireland, where by tradition both the old and the young with special needs are looked after at home, cared for by their family, not hidden away in institutions. Nursing homes, or care homes, are relatively new, and some, like Ballintobber Lodge, retain the atmosphere of a family home, while of course conforming to all the rules and regulations. 'Often the bravest and most humane decision is to do nothing,' Gawande says of end-of-life care. I had already agreed to a minimal-intervention plan for Aidan, and I was glad that Gawande's book reinforced this decision.

We had watched the funeral of Seamus Heaney on the big communal television on 2 September 2013. I wasn't sure that Aidan had taken it in fully, and I knew that most likely he wouldn't remember who had died. So when his great friend Dermot Healy died suddenly on 29 June 2014, I decided not to tell him. Nor did I go to the funeral – Helen assured me there was no reason to 'make the trek' – the four-hour drive to Sligo. There would be a large attendance, so I preferred to spend the time quietly with Aidan. When I arrived at Ballintobber Lodge on the day of the funeral, he greeted me with the words, 'Anything strange?', the opening line of Dermot's novel, *Fighting with Shadows*, which we had taken to using sometimes as a greeting.

Similarly when Bernard Share died, and Paulette O'Farrell, and so many other friends: it seemed better not to burden him with the sorrow. Mossie was the first cat to die, followed about a year later by Naseby, aged eighteen and nineteen. When his son Carl had a stroke on 1 January 2015 that left him paralysed on the right-hand side, it also seemed kinder not to tell Aidan. He would occasionally mention someone, his brother Colman, for example, and add, 'I suppose he's dead too?', as if it were inevitable in the way of things. And it usually was.

I drove up to Galway to meet Helen Gillard Healy at a commemorative event for Dermot on the afternoon of Saturday, 25 April 2015 as part of the Cúirt literary festival.

Helen was driving back to Sligo after, but I headed south for Kinvara, where I had decided to spend the night. I wanted to make the most of this break, and do a long-planned Yeats walk from Thoor Ballylee to Coole Park the next day before heading home.

I was in the car by 10.30 the next morning, changing into my walking boots, when the phone rang. It was Abby from Ballintobber Lodge to say that Aidan had had a bad turn in the night, and was in the resuscitation unit at Cork University Hospital. They had been ringing my landline earlier, and got no reply. I put my shoes back on, and drove non-stop to Cork, arriving at 1.15 p.m.

By the time I got there, they had moved him out of the resuscitation unit and onto a trolley in the corridor, while waiting for a bed to be ready, which was the default mode in Irish Accident & Emergency wards. The nurse said getting a bed could take until the small hours, or even tomorrow. I was sure he was on the mend; he looked much as usual, but very tired. Then I wondered if I had my head in the sand: was it more serious than I thought? I read a proof copy of Dermot Healy's new *Collected Stories* as I sat with him, the perfect book to be absorbed in, even if it did raise the hairs on the back of my neck all the way. Dermot knew his time was nearly up; he was wise beyond imagining.

I left once Aidan was asleep. I said no sentimental goodbyes because I really did believe he would be OK in the morning, just a few steps further down the hill. Down the hill to where? To the end, let's face it. Either Aidan was quietly fading away, or he was facing into a new phase of greater discomfort, being fed a liquidised diet, unable to walk independently, and all that goes with that.

I had requested no high-tech interventions, but I could see that it made sense for Aidan to be in CUH, in case there was anything they could do to lessen the effect of the 'turn' – most likely a stroke. He would need to be seen by speech and language therapists, and by occupationaltherapists and physiotherapists to assess his walking ability and his swallow before he was discharged.

I rang the hospital first thing in the morning, and was told he had been moved to the High Dependency Unit, a newly opened section of Accident & Emergency. I had a short wait in a sparkling new first-floor room before being shown into a large ward with one high bed in the middle of it. The body lying in it was completely swaddled in a blue hospital blanket, face covered, so that it seemed at first glance to be dead. I felt a terrible stab of grief – why had they not warned me he had died? Then I realised he was still alive, breathing heavily and perhaps frightened. I made contact, and he opened his eyes, and seemed to take in what I was saying. Tears of relief were pouring down my face. That would have been a terrible way to die, alone and frightened. I sat beside him for a while, holding his hand, and he drifted off to sleep.

The stroke had left Aidan paralysed down one side, and unable to walk. It had also affected his swallow. I was late for my first visit to Ballintobber Lodge since the stroke. I had promised to be there at 2 p.m. but didn't get there until 3, not knowing that he had been waiting for me all that time in the red wing chair in the hall. Eventually, he got fed up with waiting, and had somehow made his way up the baronial curved staircase to his old room, Room 15, in spite of being paralysed down his right side.

A staff meeting was just ending as I arrived, and I asked Raj, the new nurse manager, where I would find

Aidan. We were interrupted by a man with wild grey hair, a piece of paper in his hand and his tongue sticking out, who was wandering along the corridor, apparently lost and confused. He approached Raj, and held out the piece of paper: 'This is my sister's phone number, she will come and get me.' A new arrival. Then I saw Eugene, a kindly looking dementia patient who was admitted at the same time as Aidan, being escorted along the corridor by two carers, one in front, one behind, Eugene barely able to shuffle along in between them. The average length of stay in a home is three years. Eugene and Aidan are both at two years, four months.

When Raj reappeared, I asked, 'But where is Aidan?' Raj asked one of the care assistants, who said Aidan was in the dining room. Another said he was in Room 10, and another said Room 6. So I went upstairs, and he was not in 10 or 6. So just in case, I had a look in Room 15, his old room at the front of the house, and there he was. The man who couldn't walk had somehow made his way up the long curved staircase and was sitting in his usual chair by the window, his bed unmade, just the rubber mattress – but his books, Matisse, *Flotsam and Jetsam* and so on, all lined up on the windowsill along with the bluebells I had brought in the previous Thursday, before leaving for Galway. It seemed like weeks ago. Now he wanted to go and lie down, but he could hardly stand, let alone walk. So I went for help.

I found Rollo, the tin whistle player, his special friend. He said he'd come up with Romeo when they had finished moving someone else, which they did. When it became apparent that Aidan couldn't walk, even with the help of two men, they decided to put him in a wheelchair and gently roll him downstairs. Romeo, a beautiful young Filipino, introduces himself to Aidan by singing 'Ave Maria', so that Aidan knows who it is.

Ave Maria, gratia plena
Maria, gratia plena, Ave, ave dominus,
Dominus tecum.

Aidan smiles at the performance, which he hears almost every day. We are joined by English Susan, a wiry, dark-haired woman in her sixties with a soothing voice and a cockney accent, and Sinead, one of the young Irishwomen working here. Between them they discuss ways of getting Aidan back downstairs so that he can lie down, as he is so obviously tired. The women think lowering the wheelchair down the curved stairs is too dangerous, but Rollo and Romeo demonstrate, and they agree it's worth trying. And while all this was going on, a silent telecoms engineer was working away on the floor under our feet, measuring out lengths of coloured cable. I reassured Aidan that he'd soon be lying down – then he was put into the wheelchair and off they went, the four carers and Aidan, with many an 'Ave Maria', until they reached the ground floor.

Rollo and Romeo put him to bed, gently removing his shoes and socks. I was struck by their kindness toward him, and the gentleness with which they handled his paralysed side – 'Good man', the chosen words of encouragement. 'Give me your arm there, good man, sit down there now, good man, good man.'

I commented on how good Rollo was at handling non-responsive patients, and asked if he had to do a lot of courses to qualify for this job?

'Yes, but you only do them for the piece of paper. I have my own ways of doing things, and once I've got the piece of paper, I stick with what I know.'

As did Romeo, the singer of 'Ave Maria'. Rollo was a musician, and only worked mid-week as his weekends were for performing.

At last Aidan was in a lovely fresh bed by the window, head on three plump pillows, and I sat beside him, hoping he'd fall asleep. I lowered the blind, and opened the window a crack to hear the birdsong. 'Good man!'

As I waited to leave at the front door (which has to be opened for me and closed after), little Alice was making her way upstairs, which I pointed out to Angela, a Filipina care assistant, who coaxed Alice back down by singing 'Ave Maria', perfectly in tune, but not as beautifully as Romeo. Philippa, the lady who comes to play cards with people in the afternoon, opened the door for me, laughing at Angela's song, and I left with 'Ave Maria' and 'Good man!' echoing in my mind.

After the stroke Aidan could no longer walk unaided. But he could stand up, and he could set off, which was dangerous, because very soon he would fall. He couldn't remember that he can't walk. He wouldn't accept it. So from then on, he would have to be kept in the place that I call 'the dementia room', a conservatory extension to the right of the home's front door, where about a dozen of the higher-dependency patients spend their days.

2 May 2015

As I arrive at the front door, and wait to be let in, I can look in and see Aidan sitting at a table. Sometimes he is staring straight ahead, the staff see me waving, and tell him I'm there, and he waves back. Other times he has his arms on the table, and his head down on his arms, and I feel sorry for the long day that he has to get through. But it is better for him to be up and dressed and sitting at a table than lying in bed all day dozing. Even so, I realise that his inability to walk probably means that he will not last much longer.

2 May 2015, In the Dementia Room

Faith of our fathers, living still,
In spite of dungeon, fire and sword;
Oh, how our hearts beat high with joy
Whene'er we hear that glorious Word!
Faith of our fathers, holy faith,
We will be true to thee til death.

Aidan's neighbour in the dementia room, on a day bed-like chair, her legs out in front of her, a small fierce-looking woman with straight steel-grey hair, belted out the above, word perfect, after lunch. She has a giant rosary (white plastic) around her neck. 'I have said my morning prayers,' she announces to the room in general.

Beastly hymn, written in 1849 by Frederick William Faber (1814–1863), a convert, who founded the London Oratory – 'Priests of the Congregation of St Philip Neri' – where sometime in the 1950s Aidan's brother Colman married Sylvia Musgrave of Greystones in a side chapel, ever modest.

'I said my morning prayers, I did!' A boastful shout from Faith of Our Fathers. I remembered one of my neighbours, an elderly Protestant, warning me that Aidan would find a very Catholic ethos at Ballintobber Lodge, not realising that we are – officially anyway – Catholics.

Bridget McFadden, the Faith of Our Fathers woman, has a permanent desire for a hot cup of tea. 'I'd like a hot cup of tea please.' She can say it twenty times in half an hour, in a 'good girl' voice that you couldn't argue with. Every so often, as is the way of things, she is given one. Then she says: 'And a sandwich, please.' The two smiling young beauties – care assistants – one blonde, one dark, in their late twenties, are standing in the midst of the dementia room, radiating goodness, proving that beauty comes from within.

11 May 2015

Email from Jonathan Williams, Aidan's agent, who had sent my story collection to Aidan's former editor, Robin Robertson, at Jonathan Cape. 'Robin Robertson has replied very quickly to say that he cannot make your collection of stories work in the current UK marketplace.' How tactful of Robin, and how kind to answer so quickly.

I am very impressed by the patience of the staff in the dementia room – Gráinne, Adrian, Reuben, Romeo, Ann, Susan the carer, Susan the nurse, and Polish Gosia. They spend their time mopping up dribble and snot, taking each one to the toilet and back, spending a few minutes keeping them cheerful, talking to them by name – 'Sit down, Tim, sit down now and stay there, good man...'

I always wondered what it was like to visit someone who was not right in the head, and not sure why you're there, or even who you are. I remember my father's friend Ashley Good, and his daily visits to his wife, and my reluctance to ask him how he did it. Well, now I know what it's like. Aidan knows me, he knows it's Alannah, his wife, but doesn't know what to do with me. He feels he should be amusing, entertain me, but he can hardly speak, cannot see, and quickly loses track of what is going on.

His son Elwin and Elwin's son Oscar, aka Ozzy, aged nineteen, came to visit, which was a welcome distraction. Aidan was thrilled to have them here, but he was sad when they left. And he was as cranky with them as he is with me, but they took it better, more philosophically. Elwin has spent years working with troubled teenagers, so he's seen it all, but Ozzy's quiet acceptance of a potentially very upsetting situation impressed me. Because Aidan is their father/grandfather, he is allowed to get old.

Now when I visit, at first he is glad to see me, and he smiles and takes my hand in his so-familiar one. We are friends for about twenty minutes, then he turns, and starts trying to manipulate me to help him get out of there, to let him walk upstairs to his old room, to take him away from here altogether. Then the carers see how it is going, and help me to slip away while they distract him.

From outside the room, in the car park, I see him staring blindly around him, moving his head as he 'looks' for me with his sense of hearing, touch and smell, and my heart breaks – so I must still love him in some way. All too often I drive away in tears – and I wonder why I'm finding life hard, and not writing enough, nor reading enough, and needing treats and breaks. I have a residency at Cill Rialaig, an artists' retreat on a clifftop in Kerry, coming up in August, ten whole days in a cottage by the sea, to write uninterrupted. The prospect helps to keep me going. I can come home halfway through and visit Aidan, and friends will visit while I'm away and keep him entertained. It will happen if I want it to.

Meanwhile, I escaped to Lismore for the weekend, Immrama Travel Writing Festival, civilised company in a civilised place, including my good friend and colleague Paul Clements from Belfast, and the historian Turtle Bunbury, whom I've wanted to meet for ages. On my way home I stopped in at Glencairn Abbey for sext, the nuns singing their office in their sunlit church. Half an hour of heavenly therapy. It's amazing what consolation is there once you start looking for it.

9 June 2015

I got to Ballintobber Lodge at 2.45, and through the window as I waited for the front door to be opened, I could see Aidan apparently uncomfortably asleep, his arm on the table and his head on his elbow. When I got to him, I bent down so that my head was at the same odd angle, looking at him face to face, was rewarded with the most lovely smile and the old eyes lighting up: 'It's you!' Whether he said it or not, that's what he meant. We held hands on top of the table, and I tried to keep my head low enough to keep looking into his eyes. They are still the same colour as my eyes, it was one of the things we noticed about each other when we first met. We were connecting through our eyes and hands more directly than through speech. After a while he started saying 'Thank you for coming...' but couldn't finish the sentence so I said 'To visit you?' and he said yes, and nodded, and I smiled and said 'It's a pleasure,' and squeezed his hands.

For the first time since the stroke, we had a good goodbye. I told him gently that I had to go now, and slid my hands out of his and kissed his forehead. Then he grabbed my hand back, and I said again, 'See you very soon,' and slipped it out of his. I left peacefully, and he straight away seemed to nod off, head on hands spread out on table. I am almost as sad at this nice farewell, which reminds me of how we used to be, as I have been at some of the rougher ones.

24 June 2015

I was woken by a call in the night, Aidan's chest infection had got worse, and the duty GP suggested that he be taken up to CUH for assessment, in case there is something they can do to help him. If there is the possibility that they can do something to help him, how can I say no?

I went up at midday, he was still on a trolley in a corridor of A&E. He had responded well to oxygen, and did not seem uncomfortable. He explained to me that the worst was that he couldn't think clearly – it was impossible to think. He looked puzzled rather than distressed at this discovery. We held all four hands in a heap and looked closely into each other's eyes. As he held on to my hands he told me (getting the words out with difficulty, but not as great a difficulty as usual) that he had believed he would never see me again, and I have an inkling, only an inkling of how terrifying that must have been, to be in strange surroundings, among strange people, with painful lungs, believing that this was the end.

The next day Aidan had been moved to a new wing. I was put to wait in a shiny new anteroom, until a nurse came and led me to him. While I stood there his doctor, a youngish man, joined me, and we had the strangest conversation. He said, 'You're a lot younger than him, aren't you?' and I said yes, twenty-three years. He told me his wife was eighteen years older than him, and asked, 'Is it difficult?'

'Yes, it's tough all right. But I wouldn't have it any other way. I had to take a chance, no one could have stopped me.'

'That's exactly what I feel, I'm glad you said that. Good luck.'

I never saw him again.

26 June 2015

I went out for a pub lunch, and when I came back Aidan was in a different bed, in a sunny corner room. He seemed well settled, so I decided that I would go as planned to the opening concert of the West Cork Chamber Music Festival. Not happily, but I am told I must keep my life going, and not be totally subsumed in Aidan's failing health.

So here I am, an hour and a half later, sitting on an embroidered duvet cover in a nice B&B on the Sheep's Head, looking out over the blue water of Dunmanus Bay, about to get dressed for a concert in Bantry House – a Mozart Quartet, then Barry Douglas playing Schubert. But still there is this conflict – should I be here, or should I have stayed with him?

I used to tell myself that I cannot go on living my life as if Aidan is going to die tomorrow – but now the possibility is far more likely – far closer – so should I stick at home and visit him more often?

No. He is in full-time care, being looked after by other people. Often seeing me only upsets and disorients him. And having experienced the kindness and expertise of his carers in CUH, I do not think it is such a bad thing if he should die in hospital. I was furious at the possibility on Wednesday, now on Friday, four visits later, I believe he could be gently eased on his way if that were the kindest thing to do.

But not just yet please. Other impossible considerations – the eyes of the old man looking up at me today, just as he looked up in that striking *Irish Times* photo from 1985 with the granny glasses and long beard – do I still love the same man? Who is he now? If anything I'd say he's a nicer man now than he was then, humbler and more kind, dementia permitting.

4 July 2015

I am glad that his good qualities are showing in his decline, his enjoyment of the scent of the lavender and rose nosegay that I brought him today from the garden – hence the word, nosegay? Check etymology.

On Compass Hill

Why do I keep moving around, compulsively travelling, whenever I can? Because I shouldn't?

At worst, one is in motion; and at best,
Reaching no absolute in which to rest,
One is always nearer by not keeping still.[2]

And when I'm at home I compulsively walk the same
walk, a half-hour circuit of Compass Hill, the one
most associated with Aidan. Out of the front door,
turn right, up Rampart Lane to Blind Gate, turn left
up the hill to Ballinacubby, past the row of brightly
coloured terraced houses and the school, swing
right at the end of Winter's Hill on to Compass Hill
itself. You are heading south, and on the right is a
distant view of the Bandon River, a big wide bend
meandering upriver. For the last ten years or so,
there is a colourful jumble of housing estates down
on the marsh below, a new development, known as
Compass Quay. The marsh is still there, and beyond
it a riding school with paddocks and horses grazing
on the slope opposite. At the first big corner of the
hill, you are facing due south. On a fine day you can
see the open sea at Sandycove on the outer harbour,
and as you swing through the angle from south
to south-east there is the 'new' bridge below –
new in 1978 – connecting Kinsale to the opposite
parish of Ringrone. As you turn up to the east you
are looking directly across at a pretty little pub with
the words THE DOCK stencilled in white on its roof.
Above the terrace of fishermen's cottages known
as the World's End you pass a stone-faced modern
house called Fiddler's Well. This place became one
of Aidan's obsesssions during the last few years he
lived at home, because a suicide had been found in
the well, back in the early twentieth century, within

living memory of the older people. By coincidence, the owners of the two big new houses beyond Fiddler's Well on the crest of the hill also killed themselves, one of them by driving his car off the Old Head. Aidan has been obsessed by the idea of suicide ever since his friends Donal and Harry killed themselves.

The next big house, Dromderrig, belonged to Denis Sheehy, the auctioneer who sold us our house in Higher O'Connell Street. By the time you reach the far corner of Winter's Hill, marked by a three-storey Georgian house known as Rampart House, you are walking to the north, along the Ramparts with a view below of that part of Kinsale known as 'the flat of town'. At the end of the Ramparts, beyond the main façade of the convent building, you once again come to the Convent Steps leading down to Higher O'Connell Street, which we shorten to Higher Street. A left turn past three front doors leads you back to ours.

Again and again I walk this walk, without Aidan, but accompanied by his obsessions, and the memories of the many occasions when we walked it together, including one stormy Christmas morning with Derek Mahon when the gusts at Windy Corner were so strong the three of us had to link arms to get around it safely.

'To walk the same way is to reiterate something deep; to move through the same space the same way is a means of becoming the same person, thinking the same thoughts.'[3]

15 July 2015

I still do not like to think about funeral arrangements. Is it superstition or good manners? Then
while awake in the middle of last night, I decided
that the 'afters', or the wake, will be in Actons
Hotel, where we first met, and I stopped fretting.
A nice symmetry. No removal, no public at the
crematorium, no clergy, only friends gathering to
remember him. And music. Peter Maxwell Davies'
'A Farewell to Stromness' in an arrangement for
guitar, and maybe at the end some cheerful instru-
mental music, Nino Rota's theme from 8½, perhaps,
played loudly. Simple, unfussy, with a touch of
humour.

Matthew is visiting Aidan today so I'm not
planning to go. At last I have recognised that me
being there for Aidan is no longer necessarily the
best thing for him – for example, Romeo is better at
feeding him than I am, Sinead and Teresa are better
at cheering him up, Rollo is better at getting him in
and out of the chair – he needs practical help, and
having me there just confuses him, reminds him,
unhelpfully, of his former independent life.

Yesterday when we'd settled in peace in his
room, escaping the accordion trio playing jigs and
reels in the dementia room, he suddenly burst out,
furious, 'When am I going home?'

I hate to say it, but I have had enough.

23 July 2015

The ten-day residency at Cill Rialaig is looming
large on the horizon. What I was looking forward to as the ultimate treat has become a terrible

prospect if I can't go, and a terrible prospect if I can, another thing to worry about rather than a miraculous opportunity to have some writing time on my own.

But today I had a lovely morning at Cahirmee Horse Fair! Sun, horses everywhere of all shapes and sizes, and donkeys and horse people, young traveller women with their babies all dressed up, and a man with a box of ferrets, frightening us and making us laugh.

I spent that August from the 10th to the 20th alone in a stone cottage on top of a cliff on Bolus Head, writing, reading, thinking, walking and swimming. On Saturday the 14th I nipped back (three and a half hours) to see Aidan – and went down again on Sunday for another five days. I reworked the story collection, retitled it *The Dogs of Inishere*, and thought it was much stronger. I also spent some time thinking about writing a memoir of Aidan, the good times, the travels, the fun, but especially about all that I had learnt in the last two years-plus, since he'd been taken into care.

22 September 2015

Feeling much better after four days in England staying with my schoolfriend, Patsy, and her new husband, Richard, whom we refer to as 'the younger man', as he is four years younger than us. Patsy and I walked the dog every morning for about an hour in fields adjacent to the village (in rural Northampton), then all three of us went somewhere – a stately home and garden, the bookshop in Market Harborough, soup and sandwich lunch in a local pub, walk around the neighbouring village, Naseby (like our late cat, coincidentally), visiting the church and the big house that belonged to the Ismay family of *Titanic* fame, remembering Derek's poem, and a day trip to the birthplace of John Clare. Hard to believe when paying that we are all now senior citizens, even Richard at 61. Mildly cheered by noticing that Richard, a writer, is even worse than I am at getting down to it (writing) – his hours of photography, piano-playing and gardening all successful displacement activities. Mine are reading the *TLS*, reading poetry, walking or swimming, gardening, lying in bed late ... we are all human.

Saturday 24 October 2015

It was a grey autumn Sunday, and I was planning to tidy the garden before the weather got worse when Abby of Ballintobber Lodge rang to ask if I could come down and help to calm Aidan. This had never happened before in all the time – almost three years – that he had been there.

Aidan was at his table, very poorly, a little feverish I thought, on antibiotics for a urinary tract infection, trying to say something. Then he got it out, slowly, deliberately and with terrible anger: 'What do I have to do to get out of here?' Abby told me he had been asking the same question at intervals for the past two days, in a state of heightened rage: 'What do I have to do to get out of here?' As if he has suddenly become lucid, and woken up to find himself trapped in this place.

Later I learn that dementia patients do sometimes have periods of lucidity when they appear to 'wake up' from their demented state to a

rational one, and cannot understand why they are
in a home. That is one of the most terrifying things
I have ever heard. I cannot even begin to imagine
how horrific it must feel, to wake up and find
yourself imprisoned in a totally unfamiliar place,
which is apparently your home.

I met Helen again, this time in Dublin, for the launch of
Dermot's *Collected Short Stories* and a re-issue of his 1984
novel, *Fighting with Shadows*. It was a Dalkey Archive event,
and Helen and I sat on either side of John O'Brien in the
front row. Anne Enright said an interesting thing about
DH's use of dialogue: 'He didn't make things up; he took
things down.'

Neil Jordan gave one of the launch speeches, and quoted
Aidan's 'very cranky' reader's report for David Marcus on
Dermot when judging the Hennessy award: 'None of the
other writers showed any sense of humour, Dermot Healy
should get first, second and third prizes.' Keith Hopper
looked gorgeous with long silver hair in a ponytail. The
writer and actor Pauline McLynn, who is Keith's cousin,
read very well, and also very generously picked up the tab
for the wine (lots) at the tapas bar we went to afterwards.
I really enjoyed the evening, and was surprised that I had
all these relatively new friends. Neil Murphy was just off
a flight from Singapore. He suggested submitting my
story collection to Dalkey Archive. Would it not look a bit
incestuous, Dalkey being Aidan's publisher? Meanwhile the
stories are doing nothing, waiting to be read by two English
publishers. Ask and thou shalt receive. I decided to email
John O'Brien about my story collection. He replied by
return, said send it along, and promised to have an answer
for me within three weeks.

3 November 2015

Lovely festive afternoon at UCC yesterday to celebrate an Hon. DLitt awarded to my friend, mathematician and biographer of George Boole, Des MacHale. We were all dressed up at 4 p.m., sitting in the Aula Max for four honorary conferrals, awaiting the speakers. It reminded me of Aidan's conferral as Hon. DLitt on 11 May 2001. Fourteen years ago, how much longer it seems, and how far away. He was not happy about it, I never found out why.

I've just agreed to edit an anthology of Cork city in poems and songs for The Collins Press. The poet George Harding, who was also at the conferral, offered to help: he has a big library of Cork-related books. 'Who's editing it?' he asked, having not been listening. '*Mé féin*.' I said (I am learning Irish). I enjoyed that.

I found an old photocopy of Heinrich von Kleist's essay 'On the Marionette Theatre', about puppeteering, and read it to Aidan. He was fascinated by it, enraptured even, something like his old self, it was lovely to see. He knew the essay well, from his days as a puppeteer, a very good one, by all accounts. Two days later he seemed to have trouble hearing or understanding me, and was all hunched over to one side in a wheelchair. I tried to talk, but he wasn't responding. I asked if anything hurt, and he balled up in rage and shouted 'Everything hurts!'

Today he was dozing in and out of consciousness, head on table, in the dementia room, which was quiet for once. He held my hands in between his to try and warm them up. He always finds my hands cold. Then he dozed off, consciousness coming and going, and did not notice when I left. All the carers are tactfully trying to make sure I realise that this is a major decline from which people of his age do not come back.

17 November 2015
Summoned to the surgery. Micheál wanted to talk to me. After listening to what he had to say, I came out with 'Let nature take its course'. Where do these words come from? But it was so right. He wanted me to know that effectively Aidan is now in palliative care and he will be allowed gently to fade away. I think I said, yes, let him gently fade away. But isn't it nicer, if more euphemistic, to say 'Let nature take its course'?

Thank God for good GPs like Micheál, and may Aidan go gently. The fading in and out of consciousness is in itself a blessing, reducing the pain of going back to the nothingness from which we came by lessening his awareness of it. As Beckett had it, 'This time, then once more I think, then perhaps a last time, then I think it'll be over, with that world too.'[4]

23 November 2015
So hard to write, but Aidan seems to be nearing the end, and seems to know it. Yesterday was bad – 'I don't want to go first' – and clinging to me. Showed him Colman's self-portrait, the little framed drawing. 'Has he gone?' he asks. And later, very sadly, 'I let him down,' all spoken with great effort.

The loveliest sight today – it was the fiftieth wedding anniversary of Monica, a dementia patient, and a bouquet of roses and lilies was delivered with a card. Sinead, the tall, dark-haired young one, and Teresa, a pretty young woman with curly blonde hair, were commenting to each other, 'Fifty years married!' and looks of wonder exchanged that turned into the most lovely wide smiles, and they walked down the dementia ward together, arm in arm, laughing, a sight more beautiful than anything in the Rose of Tralee, lovelier than roses, they were, with their warm smiling faces amid all the decrepitude.

How long will it take? Nobody knows, I'd guess a couple of weeks, but it is anyone's guess. Death is so huge, awesome and frightening. As is the reminder that this is where we're all going, this is how it will end for all of us, the one thing we all have in common, but that we never discuss.

The last time Aidan was really conscious was the day I read him Kleist's essay on marionettes, two weeks ago. The next day he was too weak to be moved, and so it went on, short visits, hand holding, and a new one, forehead rubbing. He nodded off while I sat there. By arriving a bit earlier, 2.15 p.m. instead of 3.30 p.m., I found he was more alert. I read him a few pages of Alan Bennett's *The Lady in the Van* – he remembered Alan Bennett, but not the van lady, and he was delighted. Did he say, 'I am transported'? Or did I dream it? And the rest of the dementia room was listening in, Eily, the young one of unsound mind, and big Mary Barry liking it, the pious Bridget McFadden not. Ironic to remember us both many years ago reading Alan Bennett's memoir of his mother losing her memory. They are sitting on a bench above the sea, and she asks him, 'What's the name of that thing that you go around in all alone?' and the answer is 'Car'. How we laughed...

Because he was in such good form again I read him another piece by Alan Bennett beginning, 'It is said of Robert Lowell that when he regularly went off his head...' and there was a loud shout from Eily in the corner: 'Off his rocker! He went off his rocker!' and Bridget McFadden said, 'You'd be better off saying your prayers. Our Father who art in heaven...' in that particular churchy monotone of those of her generation intent on being seen to be saintly.

It was all quite jolly all of a sudden, a communal event!

4 December 2015
I find Aidan tired and sleepy, head down on his arms on the table in front of him. I wake him very gently; he seems to recognise me. I talk to him for a few minutes, then he asks 'Are you going to give me communion?'

He has a hot forehead, slight cough, nods off again. I fear I will not see him many times more. I tell him stories, often made up. I tell him stories about the cats, Mossie and Naseby, as if they were still alive, and he smiles and likes it.

14 December 2015
I was told Aidan was in the day room, and looked along a line of old faces, some of them nutcrackers, chin and nose almost meeting, but did not see Aidan. Then I noticed a small figure in navy blue who'd slipped down the chair, eyes closed, and it was Aidan,

up and dressed, but barely able to hold himself upright. He made his 'very pleased to see me' face, but looked desperately tired and weak. The carers made room for me on an upright chair. This was the high-dependency corner, everything these patients drink must be logged. I sat by Aidan, who was being fed thickened Ribena. Unthinking, I took a swig from my water bottle, and he made a grab for it. That is what he wanted, a drink of water. But he was not allowed to have one, because he would choke, which had just happened with the Ribena, twice. The dementia. He asked to go to bed.

I woke in the night with three words burning into my mind, 'Aidan is dying'. If that is what must happen, I wish it would happen more quickly and with less distress for him. For his own sake, to ease his suffering, you could say I wish him dead. I wish it was over for him, the thirst, the discomfort, the look I see in his eyes that says 'I'm losing' – the battle for life.

I have two moods, one very bad, in which I've had enough: three years of Ballintobber Lodge visits, preceded by ten years of high anxiety and hospital corridors, and seldom any thanks from the object of all this care. And the other mood, which is grieving – for the man he once was, the man I loved and married, the man who made me feel loved and appreciated. Though that man is long departed, only traces remain, but I still miss him, and I am sad it's turned out like this.

24 December, Airport Hotel, Croydon
Can it be possible I haven't written here since 14 December? Ten whole days. And here I am in outer

London, about to spend Christmas with my brother and his family, returning home on Stephen's Day, as I now call it. 'Go, and don't feel guilty,' I was told this morning by Aidan's GP, Micheál.

Aidan came back, he almost shook off the chest infection and certainly got rid of the fever, but has since gone further downhill. He has only a few good hours a day. He tires easily, and mentally he comes and goes, though it is probably also sheer fatigue. His heart is not good, and it often seems too much effort for him to stay awake. The nurses and Nelly tell me it's very hard to get him to swallow anything now, the reflex is so weak, but he appears willing, so they keep trying. On the better days they can get him to take a couple of beakers, but some days he gets no nourishment.

I sit and hold his hand and make him as comfortable as possible. It is painful to see him, the thin bones, all shrunken. He likes to lie facing the wall, with his good left hand crossing his body to hold on to the edge of the mattress. This morning when I woke in an unfamliar single hotel bed, I found myself taking that position too, unconsciously. It made me feel more anchored, tied down by my own limbs.

I only hope the diminishing of his senses makes it easier for him, less intense. His sight is almost gone, hearing low, smell who knows, taste? He still has enough to dislike some liquid foods, but definitely touch is still the strongest sense of all. He still enjoys holding my hand, and I like to hold his, as I always have done, but very gently. My hope is that with less active senses, he suffers less: time passes, one day elides into another, the faces around him are familiar, as are the voices and the contact. Then he is taken back to his quiet bed, fresh sheets, a triangle of plump pillows.

Micheál has been the best possible support to both of us. Last week he asked me to come and see him in the surgery again. In spite of a packed waiting room, he sat me down and said he'd noticed another big decline, and he didn't think there was much more that could be done other than to make Aidan as comfortable as possible, and was I okay with this? I said he was thirsty, was there any way he could be hydrated, a drip perhaps? Micheál explained that this was not considered good practice, as it was only a temporary respite, but he could tell the nursing staff to let him sip a little unthickened water if he wanted to. I thought that was a great idea, even at the risk of him aspirating some. Then as if talking to himself, Micheál said it would be a good idea to get the hospice team down to look at him, and advise. His medication is so complex, and they are used to dealing with this. That made it seem so final, tears started pouring down my face and he had to give me a paper towel. I started thanking him and that only made it worse, but I managed to say, 'You've been amazing, all the way along, thank you so much,' which only made the tears worse again – so I left, damply.

I saw Aidan that evening, Tuesday 22nd, around 5 p.m. He was sleepy so I let him doze. While I was there English Susan and Muntoj came in to say goodbye, as they were going off shift until Monday, which I thought was very nice of them, beyond the call of duty. Micheál said the carers found this stage very difficult because they get fond of the people they look after over the years. Susan asked me how long he'd been there, and I said three years, almost to the day, it was 21 December when he went in back in 2012. He was there for all of 2013, all of 2014, and up to this point in 2015. The sunny first-floor room, the entreaties to be let out, the sweet welcomes I had, the lovely smile and hug, good days, bad days, so many days. But no release for him, only the final one, getting ever nearer.

I told Micheál I had booked to go to London from Tuesday afternoon to Saturday for 'the Christmas', but was thinking of changing my plans. He said, 'There is absolutely no reason why you shouldn't go, and you mustn't feel guilty about it, there is nothing you can do here. Go without guilt.' Did he really say that? Well, that's what I remember hearing, as I stood in the corridor of the surgery, saying goodbye.

I called in to Ballintobber Lodge on my way to the airport and it was one of the best visits since his early December crisis. Aidan knew me, and we rubbed foreheads as we sat at the table, and I got a lovely smile, eyes and all. I gave him Tomi Ungerer's Christmas card, and he repeated 'Tomi', and looked at it smiling. We held hands and I told him bits of news and stayed half an hour. As usual, the care assistants helped me to disappear quietly, and Rollo let me out. I was in floods of tears again, as he said, anticipating the inevitable, 'I've been through it twice myself,' and he repeated what he had said just before: 'We fought like cats and dogs, but I'm very fond of him.'

Now when Aidan gets confused he calls 'Mama! Mama!', and it is me he is looking for, not his mother, Lil. The name (Jill? Alannah? Zinnia?) escapes him (he has called me all three at random over the last three years), but he remembers the sentiment. Mama! Mama! Can we call it love? That is what it feels like.

While I've been watching Aidan slowly fade away, I've been wondering, to what extent do we invent the person we love, and to what extent do we really love the other? Am I so sad because Aidan is not the lover I created in my mind any more, or am I so sad because the man everyone – including me – knew, is no longer himself? Has he gone, even before dying? If it were an elderly relation I was observing – father, grandfather, uncle – it would not be as painfully sad, because it was not a relationship based (initially at least) on romantic love – the girl meets boy thing – or youngish woman (37) meets brilliant man still in his prime (59) and discovers both a lover and a soulmate, the person she most wants to spend time with, share her life with. Until he starts to change, to be someone else, an other. I can trace that to a precise moment, late lunchtime on a sunny October day in an old-fashioned bar in New York – but that is *scéal eile* (another story).

25 December 2015

My brother and his wife have a traditional Christmas Day drinks party for their friends and neighbours. There are thirty people for drinks, and fourteen, all family, for lunch after, enough people to allow me to forget, for a little while at least, the terrible sadness of Aidan fading. I was standing in a group in the kitchen, sipping champagne, nibbling on smoked salmon, discussing the midnight Mass. My brother and his wife, and some of the people here, sing in the church choir. Someone asks what we thought of the long church service the night before. I keep quiet out of politeness, because I am a guest here, and my brother and his wife are devout Catholics. Another man in the group, an ex-Catholic like me, currently living abroad, who was there because he was staying with his equally devout sister, gave his verdict: 'Excruciating, especially the bishop's sermon.'

He used exactly the word I would have used, excruciating, which made me smile, and he picked on the part I most disliked, the bishop's pompous sermon. We got talking, both praising how genuinely multi-cultural this part of south London, including the church congregation, had become in the course of our lifetimes, vehemently agreeing about what a good thing that is. Against all the odds, I was enjoying myself, having, at least on the surface, a happy Christmas. Then I realised there is something very attractive about a like-minded man; it was as if a streak of light had suddenly entered my life. It was a hint, a kind of premonition, that there might be more moments like this in life after Aidan, other people, even perhaps a lover, with whom I could have a strong rapport.

We had finished eating and were playing word games when Micheál rang from Ballintobber Lodge. He wanted to warn me that Aidan had deteriorated, but would most likely last another day or so. My flight was at 4.35 the next day; I would be with him soon after 6 p.m. There was no earlier flight. I knew when I decided to go to London that I was risking not being there for the end, and I had chosen to take the risk, somehow knowing, however odd it sounds, that Aidan wouldn't leave without saying goodbye to me.

I drove straight from the airport to Ballintobber Lodge. Nelly opened the door and gave me a gentle hug, saying 'Thank God you got here in time.' Aidan was in bed alone in his room, with soft lighting and the curtains drawn. Nelly drew up a chair for me, and I took his hand. He squeezed it in response to my touch, and whispered 'Zin'. Yes, I had got there in time. Everything was going to be all right.

Every few hours Nelly and the Polish care assistant, Gosia, came in to turn Aidan and make him comfortable. While they were doing this I went and made a cup of tea and a slice of toast in the kitchen.

And so the hours passed, slowly and peacefully. Around 2 a.m. his breathing got lighter, and his hand lost its grip. Around 4 a.m., almost imperceptibly, his breathing stopped, and I realised that I was alone in the room. I kissed him one last time on the forehead, and went to open the window. Then I went to tell Nelly and Gosia he had gone. 'I'm so glad you opened the window,' said Gosia. 'We do that too in Poland, we always open the window.'

27 December 2015
Home in bed in Higher Street.

So ends a life. Or does it? When did Aidan die? My Aidan. Fourteen years ago, or an hour and a half ago? How strange is time when it comes to death. And how beautiful death can be when it comes with peace and gives a gentle release.

Rest in peace, my beloved.

AFTERWORD

I was escorted home in the dark by one of the young carers from Ballintobber Lodge, who drove behind me in his own car to ensure that I arrived safely. He was in tears as we set out, having been fond of Aidan, and seeing his distress set me off too. But we made it safely, and he saw me in the door.

I spent the next few weeks in a state of great relief, glad that Aidan had died so peacefully, and that the terrible burden that life had become for him had been lifted. I experienced something very like the state of emotional 'thawing out' that I had been through three years earlier, when he first went into care. Gradually I started to be less frozen, to react normally to life, to do things I wanted to do without feeling guilty because Aidan was not able to join me.

By mid-February, when all the formalities had been concluded and things were back to normal, I decided I needed a break. I wanted to go somewhere new, but I didn't want to travel very far. Eventually I opted for a long weekend in Liverpool, which my friends found hard to understand. Why Liverpool? Well, mainly because there was a direct flight from Cork, and Liverpool was somewhere I had always wanted to visit. My architect uncle Cecil Elsom had told me it was one of the most interesting cities in England for its port buildings, its two modern cathedrals and its municipal art collection. A young Mexican had recently told me that of all the excursions he had taken during a year in Oxford, his favourite was Liverpool and the Beatles' Magical Mystery Tour. Malcolm Lowry was born just across the Mersey on the Wirral, and I'd never been there either.

So it was that on a cold Saturday afternoon I found myself lounging in my hotel room, with a view of the Mersey, while watching the National Hunt racing on TV and gossiping on the phone with Eileen Battersby, trying yet again to explain why I had chosen to be in Liverpool. I had a ticket for the Magical Mystery Tour the next day, and on Monday I was taking a train to West Kirby to visit Malcolm Lowry's childhood home, returning via Port Sunlight. It was the sort of outing that Aidan would have hated, but he would have loved hearing me tell him about it.

It was the start of my life without Aidan.

Ussy sur Marne
Sept. 17 1951

dear mr Higgins
Thank you for your letter of aug. 18th .
    I don't remember what it is you can't read. I can't type this letter, being in the country without typewriter. I can't write any or won't write any more legibly than this.
    As I explained to John, I have only one copy of <u>watt</u> *and can't part with it. There is little chance of its ever being published. Another extract will appear in December issue of* <u>Irish Writing</u>.
    If I ever have the energy to make other copies I'll send one to John since he wants one, and then to you.
    If he said the millionth time I suppose he meant in his turn, after the million others.
    I could not help you from beyond help to beyond help. Not never. So better not consult me. Despair young and never look back. In the National library, gallery or elsewhere. The cherry orchard. For wisdom see Arland Ussher, 14 Strand road, merrion.
Wishing you well
Sam Beckett

ACKNOWLEDGEMENTS

Thanks to Carl, Julien and Elwin Higgins, Aidan's sons, for agreeing to this project, and to Elwin for much practical help over the years, cheerfully given, and the useful background in his book *Patches of Time* (Amazon, 2017). And to Fiona Adamczewski, Aidan's oldest friend, for many fascinating insights into his world.

Thanks to Jonathan Williams, literary agent and editor, for looking after Aidan's work over the years, and sometimes mine.

To Stephen Enniss, Director of the Harry Ransom Center, University of Texas, for a Fellowship that enabled me to spend time reading Aidan's papers in Austin in March 2019.

To John O'Brien of Dalkey Archive Press, for his enthusiasm for Aidan's work, unabated since 1983. To Edwin Higel of New Island Books, for the Dublin editions of Aidan's work, and for taking on this project.

To Neil Murphy for all he has done for Aidan over the years, and for much kindness and encouragement. To Neil Donnelly, writer and director of the Higgins documentary *Where Would You Like the Bullet?* (2018), director of the 'Aidan Higgins at 80' festival in Celbridge, County Kildare in 2007, and my guide to Celbridge in 2019.

To Peter Murray for permission to use his piece on the Trinity reading, and many helpful conversations; Suzy O'Mullane for permission to use her account of the portrait painting; Matthew Geden for his piece on reading to Aidan; and Augustus Young for 'Poem 100' from his *Dánta Grada* (Menard Press – Advent Books, London, 1975).

To Mr David Inglesby FRCOphth, ophthalmic surgeon, for his explanation of Aidan's eye trouble, and Dr Barry Ó Muirithe MRCPsych, geriatric psychiatrist, for insights into Aidan's psychiatric history.

To Liam Ronayne, Cork City Librarian, the poet Thomas McCarthy and Francis Humphrys, Director of West Cork Music, for events in Cork and Bantry featuring Aidan's work.

To Noelle Campbell Sharpe for residencies in Cill Rialaig in August 2015, February 2016 and August 2020 that facilitated work on my stories and this project.

To my brother Denis and his wife, Jenny, my sister Pixie, my niece Gabriela and all the friends who kept me sane through good times and bad, especially Katherine and Joachim Beug, Carlo Gébler, Matthew Geden, Helen M. Gillard, Hilary Hale, Philip and Patsy Harvey, Richard and Patsy Hollingum, Sarah Iremonger, Derek Mahon, Peter Murray, Vivienne Roche, Gemma Tipton, Denyse Woods, Gerry and Marcia Wrixon and John Young.

To Clíodhna Ní Anluain, who included an early draft of 'The Thunderbolt' in *Miscellany 50* (New Island and RTÉ, Dublin, 2019), and Jake Regan, who included 'Bloomsday', an excerpt from an early draft, in the anthology *The Globe and Scales* (Marrowbone Books, Dublin, 2020).

Thanks to Bill Swainson, for his consistent support for Aidan's work since the John Calder days back in the 1970s, and for agreeing to edit this book. And my thanks to all at New Island Books, especially commissioning editor, Aoife K. Walsh, who kept an eagle eye on everything.

NOTES

PART I: The Thunderbolt 1986–88

[1] James Knowlson, *Damned to Fame: The Life of Samuel Beckett* (London: Bloomsbury, 1996), pp. 6–7.

[2] Aidan Higgins, *Helsingør Station & Other Departures: Fictions & Autobiographies 1956–1989* (London: Secker & Warburg, London 1989).

[3] Alannah Hopkin, *The Dogs of Inishere* (Victoria, TX: Dalkey Archive Press, 2017).

[4] Aidan Higgins, *The Whole Hog* (London: Secker & Warburg, 2000), pp. 12–13.

[5] Aidan Higgins, *Balcony of Europe* (London: Calder and Boyars, 1972), p. 451.

[6] Ibid., p. 15.

[7] Aidan Higgins, *Donkey's Years* (London: Secker & Warburg, 1995), p. 280.

[8] *The Irish Times*, 17 June 1988.

[9] Letter from Aidan Higgins to Robin Robertson, 14 November 1987, Harry Ransom Center (hereafter HRC).

PART II: A Very Long Honeymoon 1989–98

[1] 'The Missing Link', *The Fragility of Form*, Ed. Neil Murphy (Champagne, IL and London: Dalkey Archive Press, 2010).

[2] Aidan Higgins, *March Hares* (Victoria, TX: Dalkey Archive Press, 2017), p. 286.

[3] Samuel Beckett quoted in Alec Reid, 'The Reluctant Prizeman', *The Arts*, November 1969, p. 63.

[4] 'Buffer Zone', review of *Tomi: A Childhood Under the Nazis* (London: Roberts Rinehart Publishers, 1998).

[5] Jill Anders, *McDaid's Wife* (London: Marion Boyars, 1988).

[6] Aidan Higgins, *Lions of the Grunewald* (London: Secker & Warburg, 1993), p. 125.

[7] Gerry Dukes, 'Life with the Lions', *Irish Times*, 13 November 1993.

[8] Aidan Higgins, Diary, 2 November 1993, HRC.

[9] *Donkey's Years*, p. 323.

[10] *Cara*, September–October, 1986

[11] Bernard Share, 'Auld Lang Rish and After' in *The Fragility of Form* (Champaign, IL and London: Dalkey Archive Press, 2010), p. 63.

[12] *Donkey's Years*, p. 16.

[13] Donovan Wylie, *32 Counties: Photographs of Ireland, with new writing by thirty-two Irish writers* (London: Secker & Warburg, 1989), p. 204.

[14] Colm Tóibín, 'How to Plagiarize Yourself', *The Times Literary Supplement*, 19 January 1996.

[15] *Donkey's Years*, p. 32.

[16] Derek Mahon, 'We Shift About', *The Times Literary Supplement*, 11 May 2007.

[17] Anthony Cronin, *Samuel Beckett: The Last Modernist* (London: HarperCollins, 1996), p. 567.

[18] Aidan Higgins, 'Tribute', in *Beckett at Sixty: A Festschrift*, edited by John Calder (London: Calder and Boyars, 1967), pp. 91–2.

[19] Aidan Higgins, 'Tired Lines, or Tales my Mother Told me' in *A Bash in the Tunnel: James Joyce and the Irish*, edited by John Ryan (Brighton: Clifton Books, 1970), pp. 55–60.

[20] *Samuel Beckett: Photographs by John Minihan*, with an introduction by Aidan Higgins (London: Secker & Warburg, 1995), p. 3.

[21] Ibid., pp. 8–9.

[22] Ibid., p. 9.

[23] Ibid., p. 13.

[24] Ibid., pp. 20–1.

[25] *March Hares*, p. 19.

[26] Letter from Derek Mahon to Aidan Higgins, 1995, HRC, transcribed into Aidan's diary for that year.

[27] C. L. Dallat, 'Decline in the West', *The Times Literary Supplement*, 21 March, 1997.

[28] Aidan Higgins, *Dog Days*, p. 271.

[29] Ibid., pp. 71–2.

[30] C. L. Dallat, 'Rory of the Hills Returns', *The Times Literary Supplement*, 3 April 1998.

PART III: 'A Surly Fellow of Advanced Years' 1999–2012

[1] *The Whole Hog* (London: Secker & Warburg, 2000), p. 400.

[2] Ibid., p. 399.

[3] *The Times Literary Supplement*, 29 December 2000, p. 19.

[4] Adapted from an address given by Suzy O'Mullane at Aidan's funeral, with her permission.

[5] Ibid.

[6] *The Review of Contemporary Fiction*, Vol. III, #1 William Eastlake / Aidan Higgins, Spring 1983 (John O'Brien, Elmwood Park, IL).

[7] Aidan Higgins, *Darkling Plain (Texts for the Air)*, edited by Daniel Jernigan (Champaign, IL and London: Dalkey Archive Press, 2010) and 'Discords of Good Humour: A Feature on the Life of Brian O'Nolan'.

[8] Dalkey Archive Press website, repeated in Zoom interview, 11 May 2020.

[9] Antonia Fraser, letter to Aidan Higgins, 16 February 2009.

[10] *The Whole Hog*, p. 351.

[11] *Cork Literary Review*, Vol. XIII, 2009, reprinted with permission.

[12] Peter Murray, reprinted with permission.

[13] Aidan Higgins, *Blind Man's Bluff* (Champaign, IL/ Dublin/ London: Dalkey Archive Press, 2012), p. 57

PART IV: Scenes from a Receding Life 2012–15

[1] Tomi Ungerer, *Tomi: A Childhood under the Nazis* (London: Roberts Rinehart Publishers, 1998).

[2] Thom Gunn, 'On the Move', *Collected Poems* (London: Faber, 1994).

[3] Rebecca Solnit, *Wanderlust: A History of Walking* (London: Verso, 2002), p. 68.

[4] Samuel Beckett, *Molloy*, *Trilogy* (London: John Calder Publishers Ltd., 1959), p. 8.

BOOKS BY AIDAN HIGGINS

Felo de Se: Stories [reissued as *Asylum*] (1960, 1978)
Langrishe, Go Down (1966)
Balcony of Europe (1972)
Scenes from a Receding Past (1977)
Bornholm Night-Ferry (1983)
Ronda Gorge & Other Precipices (1989)
Helsingør Station & Other Departures (1989)
Lions of the Grunewald (1993)
Donkey's Years (1995)
Flotsam & Jetsam: Collected Stories (1996)
Dog Days (1998)
The Whole Hog (2000)
A Bestiary (2004)
Windy Arbours: Collected Criticism (2006)
Balcony of Europe, edited by Neil Murphy (2010)
Darkling Plain (Texts for the Air) [radio play] (2010)
Blind Man's Bluff (2012)
March Hares (2017)